Riding The Waves During A Pandemic

Will Your Family Survive Shelter In Place Again?

Meril R. Smith

Contributing Writers

Linda Ullah

Lynn Chen

Rosanne Johnson

Israel Golden

Maria Thompson

Anthony Cedoline

RIDING THE WAVES DURING A PANDEMIC

Library of Congress Control Number:		2020910043
ISBN-13:	Paperback:	978-1-64749-135-2
	ePub:	978-1-64749-137-6
	Hardcover	978-1-64749-136-9

Printed in the United States of America

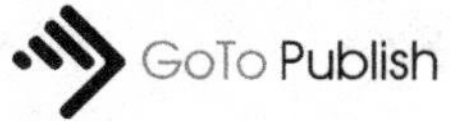

GoToPublish LLC
1-888-337-1724
www.gotopublish.com
info@gotopublish.com

DEDICATION

I have been awed and inspired
by the thousands of first responders,
health care professionals, medical support personnel,
teachers, and essential workers of all kinds,
who have put the health and safety of others
before their own.
They are true heroes in this time of pandemic.

I am also awed by the sacrifices
of the families of our heroes.
In many cases, families have not seen
their mom or a dad, wife or husband for weeks.

Finally, I am awed by the millions and millions
of families who have had to suddenly
shelter in place and whose life was
literally changed overnight.
This book is dedicated to
all families who have sheltered in place.

I May the book serve as a guide
for families who want to be better prepared,
knowing there is a strong possibility of
sheltering in place again and that more
deadly waves of this pandemic may lay ahead.

Life Lesson: *Be Safe, Wash Hands, Wear Masks and Practice Social Distancing! If you do not like wearing a mask, you are really going to hate a ventilator.*

CONTENTS

INTRODUCTION

Wash Hands, Wear Masks and Practice Social Distancing!

In mid-May 2020, reopening the United States was the big national priority. Very different ideas about Covid-19 Pandemic have become part of the way we live. Daily, we hear conflicting information. We hear the conflict between forces that put health and safety first and forces that put the need to reopen the economy first. We also hear how officials are trying to balance the two forces and come up with sensible guidelines and step-by-step procedures. The only thing we know for sure, is that we are living in a very unstable time in which information and procedures will continuously change.

There are some things of which we can almost be certain.

- New Covid-19 virus cases will continue for the foreseeable future.
- The number of new cases will depend on what happens with the development of a vaccine and the amount of testing and tracing that takes place.

- The number of new cases will also depend on what happens with how businesses and schools reopen.
- More directly the number of new cases will depend upon how each of us behaves and how seriously we take the pandemic.

The Covid-19 virus is new and scientists are learning new things about it every day. Almost all of us have been practicing personal care: washing hands frequently, wearing masks, social distancing, and sheltering in place. The things we have been doing have helped "flatten the curve" and enabled hospitals to keep from being totally swamped.

There were significant differences in how states are reducing restrictions and as businesses started the process of reopening. There are some important questions to which you may know the answer by the time you read this book.

- Did states open businesses back up too soon?
- What could happen when schools reopen and our children are back in classrooms?
- Did most people continue to wash hands, observe social distance, and continue to wear masks?
- Did we see fewer cases in the summer months?
- Since the incubation time is from 7 – 14 days, did some states see big spikes in the number of Covid-19 cases starting in June 2020?

- Will Covid-19 act similar to other pandemics: initial wave, much more deadly second wave, and less deadly third wave?

Personally, we each face a big question. Are we prepared for new spikes as well as a second and third wave of the Covid-19 virus? I do not mean medically-prepared, I mean have we actually prepared to modify the way we live and to protect our families?

Will most of us simply wait for things to happen again and then react after the fact? Will we be proactive now and make plans for harsh realities that we and our children may face? Will we have the foresight to step back from our current wants and needs in order to plan ahead? What are steps we take ahead of time, especially as it relates to our families and children? What can we do now if we end up having to shelter in place again or if schools continue distance-learning?

When the number of people being infected and the dying from the Covid-19 virus began to spiral out of control, I began thinking. Besides the medical aspects of the virus, are there other behaviors going on that may also have a significant impact on how we will live? I started reading and researching past pandemics to see what I could learn.

The first important thing that I have learned during the past months is to listen to the doctors and scientists and heed their advice. Dr. Anthony Fauci, among others, has said repeatedly that states face serious consequences if they reopen too quickly.

The second thing I learned was the need to make some simple preparations for my own family in case Covid-19 spikes or hits some areas hard and not others. There is a high probability that a second and third waves could infect hundreds of millions citizens around the world and millions of people could die?

The third thing that I have learned is the need to take better care of each other, emotionally, educationally, and interpersonally during subsequent events such as another shelter in place. We have the ability to prepare for such another event now. Will we?

The result of what I have learned – is this book! The focus is narrow...what have people done well while sheltering in place? How families decided they are not helpless victims of the pandemic? Are there steps individuals are taking to make this uncertain time a growing together and empowering experience for their family? What feelings and knowledge can we help our children take with them as they grow into adulthood? Is it possible for children to actually become better human beings as a result of this experience? I think the answer to the last question is "yes".

Background

The Covid-19 virus changed our lives almost overnight. We went from life as usual to sheltering in place, keeping distance from others, and wearing facemasks. We went from hyper patisanship politics to phoning neighbors to be sure they were alright. We went from adults going to work and kids going to school to almost everyone staying at home all day, every day. We went from our normal concerns about health to washing our hands many times each day. Although many of us have lived through mass tragedies – the World Trade Center, wars in Afghanistan and Iraq, as well as hurricanes, tornados, floods and wildfires. None of us have ever experienced anything like the Covid-19 Pandemic. As of June 2020, the United States has 5% of the world's population and 30% of the world's Covid-19 cases.

As a child, I remember hearing stories about the 1918 Pandemic. So many people were dying in Philadelphia that every morning, bodies were placed on the sidewalk and picked up by Priests in horse-drawn carts. The bodies were taken away and often buried in mass graves. In Philadelphia, 759 people died in a single day. Later, I remember reading that one third of the world's population became infected.

In 1918 there were no such things as vaccines or antibiotics. However, there were common sense public health measures. What was done in 1918 may sound a bit familiar.

- People were told to isolate themselves if they had any symptoms.
- People were told to liberally use disinfectants on surfaces to kill germs.
- People were told to practice good personal hygiene including washing hands.
- The size of public gatherings was severely limited.
- Many stores and shops were closed to prevent the spread of the virus.
- In places where there were a large number of sick people, areas were quarantined.

The measures worked well and the rate of infection slowed down by late spring. Soon people thought the worst was over and restrictions were relaxed. No one expected a second wave to hit in the fall. The second wave of the pandemic was far worse. In all, 675,000 people in the United States died and between 20 and 50 million people died worldwide.

We Have Been Here Before

In 1918, the world's population was about two billion people. About one-third of the people around the world caught the virus and between 20 and 50 million people died. In 2020, the world's population is about eight billion people. Today, the world's population is about four times as many as it was in 1918. What could the population increase mean in terms of numbers infected by Covid-19 and the number of deaths. You can do the math.

What have we learned as a society from the 1918 Pandemic? There is an old saying, "If we do not learn from history, we are bound to repeat it." With the Covid-19 Pandemic we are certainly going to find out whether or not the old saying is true?

Focus of Book

This book is not about the tragic loss of life from the Covid-19 virus or the ongoing worldwide pandemic. Rather, the book is a series of stories and observations as sheltering in place took over our daily lives in early 2020. After many weeks of sheltering in place, did we learn anything? Did we find important differences in the way we live? Did we begin to look at and treat other people a little differently? Did we change in the way we interacted within our family and community? Did we start to think about planning for our families if Covid-19 does not "magically" die out.

Through stories from parents, youngsters, teachers, and others, this book attempts to shed light on some basic thoughts.

- How did families feel about sheltering in place for many weeks?
- What kinds of strategies and activities did parents create to make sheltering in place easier?
- In what ways did the relationships change within a family?
- How were extended family members able to keep in touch...especially grandparents and grandchildren?
- What were ways people, who were sheltering in place, find to help or support others?
- How will the Covid-19 Pandemic affect the lives of individuals over the long haul?
- Is this the only wave of the Covid-19 Pandemic or will there be a second (more serious) wave and a third wave?
- As a nation, did we get a handle on Covid-19, or did our collective actions cause a renewed high rate of infection and deaths?

Wishing you thoughtful reading!

FAMILIES GROWING TOGETHER

Wash Hands, Wear Masks and Practice Social Distancing!

Weeks of "Shelter in Place" can be enough to make any family a bit "crazy." Some families have continuous upsets and hurt feelings. Other families seem to have found ways to grow together and make their family bonds tighter. These families seem to focus on finding positive ways that involve each other. Often family members play or work together, learn new ideas, create new experiences, find common interests, support each other on projects, and share chores.

This kind of thoughtful and caring approach by parents is not an accident, it is intentional. Parents model what they want to see in their children. Parents set the stage for making bonds between family members a lot stronger... especially between siblings.

Now is the time to think. What is really important to us? How can we change the way we live in ways that will help us all become better human beings?

Now is the time to plan ahead. This book is designed to help you with ideas for your own family using the experiences of others.

DID YOUR CHILD MISS SOME GRADE LEVEL SKILLS DURING SHELTER IN PLACE?

Everyone scrambled when, almost overnight, we had to shelter in place and schools closed. These were never before experiences for both adults and kids. Although teachers and schools started providing lessons within a week, it was a rocky start. Distance learning was new to teachers. Training on several distance learning programs was required. Being a new way of teaching, there were trial and error experiences. It got better as time went on. However, distance learning was certainly no substitute for children and teachers being together in a real classroom.

Some youngsters had an easy time adapting to distance learning, while many others found it difficult. I would expect that children may have a few gaps, things that were missed or they didn't completely understand.

If you feel your child had a hard time with certain skills, there are a variety of reading, language arts, and mathematics workbooks that can be used to help reinforce skills that may have been missed during distance learning. Teacher supply stores usually stock grade level workbooks. They are also available online. If you think your child may have a few gaps in one or more areas, order workbooks for the grade just completed, NOT for the new grade the child is starting.

Creating a consistent daily schedule is a must? With younger children two half hour periods and then a fifteen minute break. Older youngsters can work with your to create a schedule for them. When they are involved in creating their schedule, they are more likely to adhere to it.

An adult or older youngster needs to work with a child to help him/her understand something that was missed or very difficult. It is not necessary to use every page in the workbook. Not doing a page may be seen as a triumph of learning in the mind of a child. Your job is to find gaps that your child does not know or areas that are weak. This approach can help him/her learn and practice what was missed while they were sheltering in place and be better prepared for the coming school year.

If your child says he knows the skill on a particular workbook page, pick out a problem or question from the beginning of the page, one from the middle of the page, and one from the bottom. If your child does those three correctly, there is no need to do the entire page. Instead, praise your youngster and check out the next skill in the same way. When you find a "gap," sit with your youngster and explain the concept until the child can answer the problems or questions on his/her own. The review will help your child be much better prepared for the next grade. So relax and make it an adventure for both of you.

Educational publishers have workbooks by grade level and subject. Four publishers that you may want to review are:

- Kumon
- Scholastic
- Evan Moore
- Carson Dellosa

You may also want to check with your child's teacher for recommendations. Remember, order the workbooks for the grade level the child has just completed. That's the best way to review or reteach skills that were usually included during the time your youngsters were involved in sheltering in place. What a great way to help build your child's self-confidence!

WHAT WILL SCHOOLS BE LIKE WHEN THEY REOPEN?

As schools plan to reopen, they will not look or feel like the schools we are used to. Both parents and children will be anxious about what is happening around them and about how schooling may look like in the future.

Talking and listening to your children right now is really important. Some children may have a hard time putting their fears into words. Parents can help by sharing their concerns and asking their child(ren) simple questions. The idea that both of you have concerns or fears makes your child feel you are in this new experience together and that his/her fears are reasonable. Perhaps you have a story when you felt anxious and kept on trying until things worked out. Really listen to your child frequently. A few hugs each day and words of reassurance can really help ease anxiety.

School districts started planning months ago for this next school year. Often districts had support and guidance of the State Superintendent of Education. Covid-19 situations change quickly and it became apparent that school districts need more than one plan. The sudden spike in Covid-19 cases during July quickly changed how districts needed to plan.

The following information may be helpful as you think about how school may be different when they reopen. Students are likely to be required to wear masks. There will be a lot of hand washing. Some form of social distancing will also be implemented. Lining up, recess, and having lunch will also be different. These changes are to be expected. However, those are not the only changes that students will be experiencing. I would suggest that children practice washing hands, wearing masks, and practice social distancing every day at home. Daily practice will give your child more confidence whenever classrooms reopen and students return.

School Districts across the nation have been working hard to develop different models for educating students. Most districts also realize that if there is a large spike in the first wave of the pandemic, they may be required to change models more than once during the year. All schooling models will significantly impact parents, children and child care. The following examples are possible basic structures for schools. There is also likely to be a variety of variations within each model.

Schools Open with No Students in Classrooms:

Schools will probably not open in areas where there are significant spikes in the number of Covid-19 cases. It would be just too dangerous. Whether or not to reopen school buildings may be a state-wide decision or a county by county decision.

Distance Learning:

Despite the push to reopen all schools, there may be states or parts of states that will simply not be able to reopen. Although school districts will work to improve the Distance Learning model that was used when the pandemic first wave, Distance Learning, will probably be very similar to the one you experienced.

Distance Learning for Kindergarten through Third Grade:

The possibility of getting kindergarten through third graders to wear masks, social distance, and not share materials is a "flight of fancy" at best. Some districts may simply have these grade levels stay home and continue with distance learning. A plus of this approach is additional classrooms would be available to fourth through sixth grades, thus making social distancing easier.

Early/Late Staggered Schedules (Double Session):

Half of the class will attend the morning session and the other half will be schooled in the afternoon. Between the morning and afternoon sessions, classrooms will be disinfected. There may be a lot more learning that takes place outside on the playing fields. During the days when a child is not in class, homework packets or some type of distance learning will be used.

Two Day Rotation Blended Learning Model:

Half of the students in a class attend one day and the other half the class attends the next day. Some schools will set up cameras in each classroom, so the students at home can watch the actual lessons on days when they are not physically in the classroom.

A/B Week Rotation Blended Learning Model:

Half the students in a class come one week and the other half attend the next week. Some form of distance learning would take place on the weeks a student is not in class.

Looping Structure:

In some schools there is an opportunity for students to stay with the same teacher for a second year. Since the teacher and students already know each other, it is easier for the teacher to reteach skills and concepts with which many students are having difficulty.

Parent Option:

Some parents may feel that schools are not safe enough to protect students from Covid-19. In such cases, parents may opt to continue with distance learning programs.

The above descriptions are the simplest forms of ways to reopen schools. There may also be totally different structures. Every structure for educating students has good points and bad points. One structure may fit better in suburban areas, another one for city schools, and another one for rural schools. No matter what structure is implemented in a given school, there will be a significant adjustment for parents, students, and teachers. Don't underestimate the challenges everyone will face this next year and the following year. Again, do not be surprised if the size of the second wave of the Covid-19 pandemic requires schools to make radical changes even in the middle of a school year.

None of these descriptions take into consideration the teachers and staff. Older teachers may be at higher risk for contracting Covid-19 and may not want to teach in potentially unsafe situations.

According to Dr. Anthony Faucci, it will be at least a year before schools can get back to normal. Depending on how bad the second the third waves of the pandemic are, it may be two or three years before schools can return to normal. On the other hand, a prolonged pandemic could fundamentally change the way students are educated for the foreseeable future.

The best we can all do is to be flexible and realize that right now Covid-19 is in the driver's seat. There is still a lot to learn! Tell your children again and again that we are all experiencing new things and we are in this together as a family and we will get through this too.

An Old Memory: A New Reality (Linda Ullah)

An Old Memory

In the early 1990's my learners at Edenvale Elementary School in San Jose, California embarked on a local history project. Their goal was to write a book about the history of South San Jose. In their research, youngsters found about local Native Americans and the mysterious healing pools located in nearby hills. Research also included the first European families that settled the

Santa Clara Valley and what happened as the land became farms and ranches.

As a part of their research, youngsters found out that the first school in the area was built about 1850. Oak Grove School had a small number of students from first through eighth grade. The school was next door to a stagecoach stop, where teams of horses were switched while weary travelers quenched their thirst with cold beer. At lunch, older students would sneak over to the stagecoach stop and would return to school slightly tipsy. This lunchtime routine caused quite a stir with the wives of the local ranchers and the next year Oak Grove School was moved a half mile away.

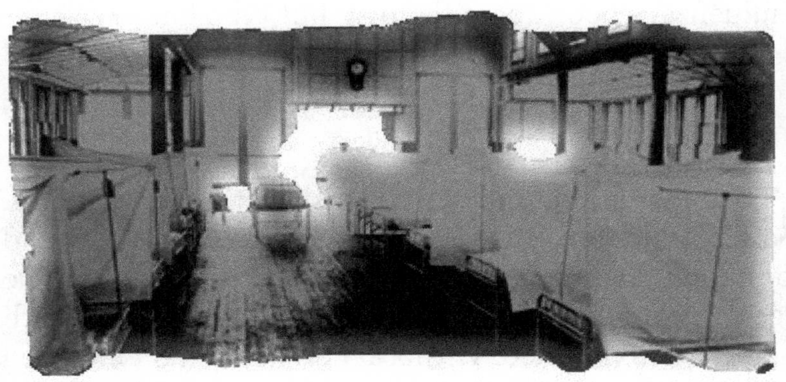

Pictures were also found of the 1881 and the 1904 Oak Grove Schools. There was an unexpected photograph of the inside of a school. What was this picture about? When was it taken? Was the school being used as a hospital? More research was required. Youngsters reviewed all sorts of information, including years of attendance registers. The big surprise came from 1918 attendance register. All the students were marked absent. A note in the attendance register said that school had been closed because of the flu. More and more information was collected and then became part of a chapter in "The Great Edenvale Detective Caper." The fifth and sixth grade students involved in writing the book had never heard of the 1918 Pandemic. Even the principal, who grew up locally, had no knowledge of this part of local history.

It is now 2020, about thirty years later. My mind flashed back to the early 1990's and the excitement we felt as we researched, discovered amazing stories, and wrote The Great Edenvale Detective Caper. I never thought about the 1918 Pandemic as anything more than long ago history and a good story. We are now in the middle of the Covid-19 Pandemic and suddenly I found myself devouring a book by John M. Barry, The Great Influenza, a book about the 1918 flu! Who knew?

A New Reality

On March 13, 2020, Jay Inslee, the Governor of Washington State announced that schools would be closed. Everyone was directed to shelter in place. The local Spokane YMCA was immediately closed, and youth sports were canceled. The local news that night included a story about the first three cases of Covid-19 in Spokane. Spokane is in the eastern part of Washington, far away from the big Seattle metropolitan area. With local cases, the Covid-19 Pandemic became real for all of us living far, far away from Seattle. The next day we began to self-quarantine. What are we going to do?

We started by going on walks and hikes just to get out of the house. Technology has helped self-quarantine easier. My sons have reconnected, via Zoom, with cousins living all over the world. Our YMCA started real time exercise classes. We also found Tai Chi videos for more home exercise. I learned to use Instacart for online grocery order and delivery.

We did Google Duo video chat with our son, Isaac, his wife, and our two year old granddaughter, Talia. For my grandson, Ethan, who lives in San Diego, we had a Zoom Birthday Party. Issac teaches at San Diego State University. Leah his wife, teaches at an alternative high school. Both are finding it very challenging to teach virtually with an active toddler scurrying around the house.

Noah, our second son, a realtor, is working virtually from home. Stephanie his wife runs a homeless "warming shelter" in downtown Spokane. Her job is high risk for Covid-19. She has not been able to come home since sheltering in place started. The two oldest boys, thirteen-year-old Ethan and eleven-year-old Logan, were rebellious about having to stay home. Seven-year-old Cohen has enjoyed playing outside. When schools were closed for the remainder of the year and virtual classes began to really hit the two older boys hard.

To curb Ethan's and Logan's anger and rebelliousness, we gave them research projects. They researched Covid-19. In addition, they did projects about two past pandemics/plagues of their choice. The projects helped them better understand why we are self-quarantining. Thankfully, their attitudes are improving. Ethan and Logan are now running two miles a day, taking hikes, and helping with household chores. It's really hard for them not to see their mother.

My son, Noah, does not really know how to cook, so both grandmothers take turns cooking dinners and leaving them on the front porch every evening. Seven year old Cohen broke my heart when he called to say he misses my hugs.

When my new glasses arrived, the optometrist's secretary brought them out and placed them on the hood of my car. When I lost a crown from a tooth and had to go to the dentist, I carried wipes and wiped down all the surfaces in the dentist's office. Twice, I have gone out to purchase plants for my garden wearing masks, rubber gloves, and taking wipes. In Spokane, we are fortunate that the few stores that are open have early morning hours reserved for senior citizens.

Our family continues to make adjustments and find new ways of surviving together. We have put our passion for traveling on hold. I am glad the Eastern Washington weather is improving and I can still garden...one of my pleasures in life. We have adjusted to a new normal. I do not know how long the pandemic will last or what life will be like. My hope is that perhaps we human beings will have become kinder and more tolerant.

Life Lesson: *No matter the results of the Covid-19 Pandemic, we will be living in a new normal. Will we go back to a highly polarized and angry country? Will we learn from the experience and realize we are all in this together? We have the opportunity to be kinder, more tolerant, and more caring of our fellow Americans.*

Sheltering = Bonding (Lynn Chen)

"Sheltering in Place", is something we are actually going through! Through my years of schooling and work, we have prepared and practiced for all sorts of emergencies. Never did we think about how to care for ourselves and others in a worldwide pandemic. Many people had never even heard the word "pandemic". "Epidemic," yes. "Pandemic," No! The Covid-19 pandemic hit us hard, very hard. "Pandemic" has become a term known around the entire world. For sure, the Covid-19 Pandemic is something that will be written in history books for our children, grandchildren and great grandchildren to learn about!

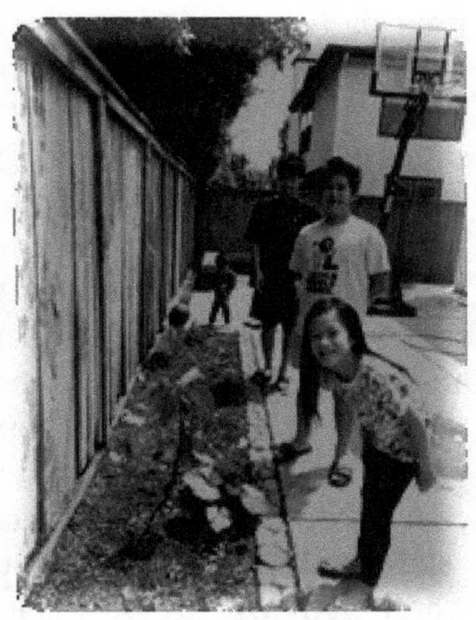

Through the Covid-19 Pandemic, some positive things did happen. As humans we usually only think of ourselves or those that are close to us. What I have learned through this ordeal is about the love and care that everyone around us has shown. It's actually true caring. We have neighbors, friends, teachers, educators, co-workers, and bosses checking in on us making sure that everyone is safe at home and taken care of. How amazing is that to see the true side of people with whom we usually don't socialize. We have created bonds by socializing more than before, however in very different and new ways.

As a family, we have documented many sides to how we function now. It's amazing to see when we go grocery-shopping and distance ourselves at least six feet from one another. It's amazing that people are only allowed to go into the grocery store a few at a time. Many shelves are empty. Toilet paper, paper towels or household products are all sold out. Masks are required and gloves are highly recommended when we have to go into a store.

What we miss most is seeing our families, my parents and siblings. It's been months since we visited relatives. What is also amazing today is we have technology to help support our daily communication with them, even from far away. There is no dining in restaurants, only take-out. One thing that has amazed me is to see how well almost everyone has integrated so many new things into their daily lives.

Kids have switched from going to school to online learning. What a new way to adapt education! What saddens me most is not seeing my eighth grader be acknowledged for his educational accomplishments or see him walk across the graduation stage. I feel for all the Seniors and Graduates who will not have a proper sendoff...senior ball, honor night, graduation ceremony, and celebrating with families and friends near and far.

It's hard knowing that our annual trips with friends will be cancelled. Our annual summer trip will also be cancelled. Mother's Day was the first time we have not celebrated with our mom's and grandmother's. It's hard when birthdays are only celebrated among the six of us. Somethings...about sheltering 24/7 is just plain hard!

What has been the most amazing part of the weeks of sheltering in place is seeing my four children bond. Their age gap has always put a distance between them. However, seeing that they are playing together in the backyard, really talking to each other and, yes, sometimes beating each other up are goals we have reached. They have bonded and really care about each other.

Finally, a picture I would like to share is the four of them getting ready to plant a garden, pulling out all the weeds, going to the stores to pick out the seeds, fertilizing the soil, and finally planting their own vegetable seeds. All four of them are awaiting the seeds to sprout. It's not about the plants. It's about the bond they are creating among each other, just like the seed hoping that one day it will sprout, grow, have flowers, produce vegetables and see them harvested and shared. What a special way to really end our family experience with this pandemic.

Life Lesson: *It is possible for four kids to bond together in ways I never imagined. And that is a very good outcome!*

Shelter in Place Experience (Rosanne Johnson)

Even as I type this, it still seems like this is all just a bad dream or like "I'm stuck in a movie." Our families world literally came to a halt weeks ago and we are still adjusting to our new normal!

Never have I wanted to homeschool my children... NEVER! My son Hunter has always wanted me to homeschool him because he says he "hates school." However, after the first few days of homeschooling Hunter kept saying, "I just want to go back to school!" Now he is finally getting his wish and he wants to go back to school. Crazy, I didn't get it! When I asked him why, he responded, "I thought being homeschooled meant you get to sleep in, only work for an hour, and then get to play and eat snacks all day!" Needless to say, this new home centered school environment was not what Hunter was anticipating.

Thankfully, all my kids have amazing schools and incredible teachers. Still I put in several hours helping them, making charts to keep them on task and organized as well as submitting assignments online. Charts are a huge help in trying to keep three kids, in three different grades, and three different school stay organized. I have a daughter who is a Junior in High School, a son who is in middle school, and a son who is in third grade. Fortunately, I also have a mom who is a teacher and who can be called upon if additional help is needed. I am happy to say that in third and seventh grade common core mathematics, "I'm killing it!" I now regret all the times I said, "I am never going to need to know how to do this math formula in real life."

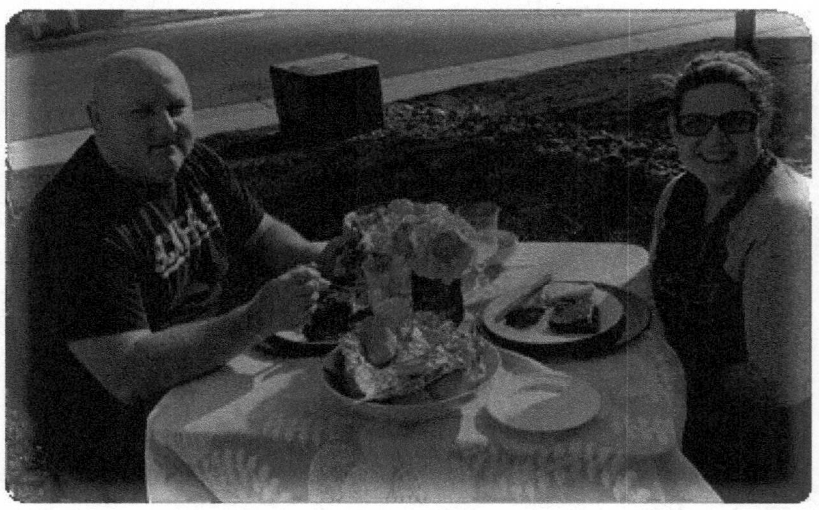

We all thrive on a schedule. The first week of shelter in place the kids didn't really have homework so I let them relax and adjust to our new life and schedule (or lack thereof). After the first week, I made an individual schedule for each kid. The schedule included when they had to be awake and up, chores, a list of every school subject and the school work that needed to be done for that day. Time was also scheduled for exercise and free time. Creating a schedule for each kid was a blessing and has made things run smoothly. I don't have to say a thing. The kids wake up, check their schedule, and get to work. Not having to nag anyone has been wonderfu...it's the new normal. I add some fun things each week such as family game nights, cooking together, family walks, and a family "Chopped" cooking challenge!

My husband and I are considered essential employees so we both still go to work. I am thankful that my kids are old enough to stay at home alone, otherwise that would be an additional hardship. My husband is in the habit of calling me on his way home and asking "What are our plans tonight?" We normally have a busy schedule with three kids involved in four different sports, so we are constantly on the go. We miss the baseball games, volleyball, flag football, and the trap tournaments. Now when my husband asks, "What are our plans tonight?" Now I say, "NOTHING!"

It felt weird as I went through our family calendar and began deleting everything. The most painful ones were deleting our plans for a huge family cruise, a trip of a lifetime, with my siblings and their families as well as plans for our anniversary...everything cancelled! We celebrated our 18th wedding anniversary, quarantine style. A card table and folding chairs were set up. I made a delicious dinner for two, complete with a table cloth and special table settings, and a romantic dinner on our front lawn. This anniversary was definitely one for the books!

At the beginning of April school was cancelled for the rest of the year and it looks like so will everything else. When I watch the news and see the devastation that Covid-19 is causing, I am grateful that we are not sick. I am grateful that my husband and I still have jobs. We are considered essential workers. I am grateful that our family is together, sheltering in one place, and that we are looking out for each other.

I am OK with 2020 when the world stopped and everything was cancelled. Years from now I will be able to say to my family, "Remember how our lives were changed and what we learned about ourselves and each other. Remember when we had to stay home all day and not play with our friends so we would not get sick or spread the deadly Covid-19 virus. Yeah, those were some CRAZY times!"

> ***Life Lesson:*** *We never know what we can really do until we are put into a very different situation. Coping sometimes take imagination and creativity. I have definitely learned that everyone in my family and my large extended family can rise to the occasion.*

"Izzy" Israel Golden

My name is Israel Golden, but I have never gone by that name. Everyone I know calls me Izzy. I am considered an essential worker. Normally I work as a Cashier at the supermarket, but right now, during these weird times, I am also the "Doorman." I keep track of how many customers that go out at the exit door or how many can be let in. I am also charged with performing a continuing headcount to make sure we are staying under our designated capacity. Why me? I worked as a bouncer in bars for 14 years and I got chosen for my experience of working with difficult people. Most customers are very nice and understanding. Every once-in-awhile someone is a real jerk and makes demands to be let into the store anyway. My job is to try to keep them calm while not letting them in. Another part is making sure each customer is wearing a mask. It's hard to understand why someone would be so crass as to put people or themselves in danger of contracting Covid-19.

With help from the Edenvale Elementary School's Adopt-A-College Scholarship Program, I am also attending San Jose City College. It took a lot of years for me to finally realize that I want and need a college education. We are using video conferencing called "Zoom" through the canvas-online app. Since the class is interactive, I must say it is closer to being in class than an ordinary online course.

My English-92 class is wonderful. I am able to communicate with my professor, Professor REW as he likes to be called, and participate in class like I normally would. With some of the scholarship money, I purchased a nice computer video and microphone system. I really appreciate to be able to take interactive classes and see my classmates as

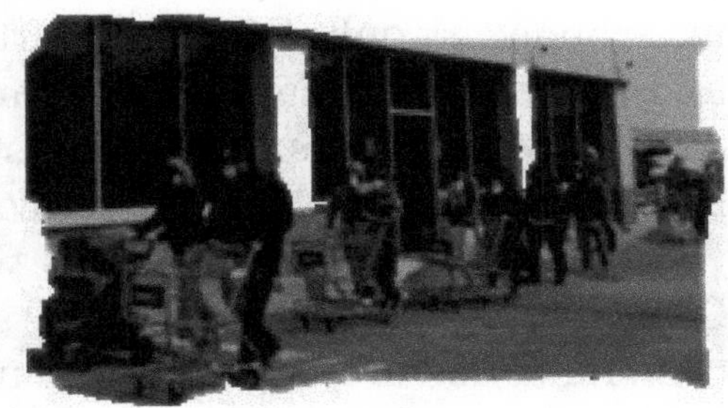

My commute to work and back is mostly by bicycle since the bus and light rail systems are now limited and

do not connect well to where I work. My life is pretty much normal because I am still working. When I am not working or commuting, I am at home doing school work, writing for my English class mainly and preparing for summer school classes.

On Tuesdays, I really miss going out and studying while I treated myself to a meal at Sweet Tomatoes. Recently, I experienced my very first college Spring Break. I had great plans that suddenly changed because of Covid-19. I really missed going to the beach. I really wanted to spend Spring Break on the ocean, surfing the waves, and relaxing. Instead I am making the most of it, by doing my English homework and writing stories. I am also rereading comic books. I am planning a way of using my new camera and microphone to read and post comic books on line so that elementary age kids can do something unique during sheltering in place.

I have found a couple of "positives" that have come out of the shelter in place order. First, I have learned more patience in helping people. Everyone is upset and stressed. People can and will take their bad day out on you if you let them. I have learned to not let customers get me down. Instead I have taken the proactive choice in being happy and helpful. It is my decision and my decision alone whether or not to be happy or unhappy. I have learned to keep other people's negativity from drowning my positivity. Secondly, I have learned to do my schoolwork online. When I started college last year, I told my counselor that I did not want to take any online courses. When I was in school last, in 1995, there was no internet in schools. I told my counselor that was the way I learn. Well, I guess I was wrong. As a result of Covid-19, my English 92 class was switched to an online conference/lecture class. I am currently doing all my courses online and that I have been able to adapt and overcome my fear of online learning.

> ***Life Lesson:*** *Some time we are surprised at the ways we can change when a life altering event happens. I am pleased that I have learned this about myself. I can adapt. I can change. It's my attitude that makes the difference.*

From A Teacher
Maria Thompson

As I received word that our school would be closed for a while, my immediate reaction was "YAY!" My first graders had been "squirmy" and had "Spring Fever", no pun intended. In my mind, a week off of school couldn't have come at a better time in the year. A couple of days before, I had sent an email home to parents. I said that I had noticed the students were having difficulty staying focused and completing work in a timely manner. However, I also said, this is the time of year we usually see this type of behavior and it is par for the course.

With a sigh of relief, I knew that the parents would have to deal with their child's spring time behavior for a few days. I truly thought of this as a welcomed break. We will be back in school soon and everything will be back to normal.

As the first week went by, I began to realize that this was not going to be as easy as I expected. The students at my school in Walnut Creek, CA were sent home with a journal and 5 library books. The first week the students were instructed to read daily and write about what they read. In addition, they were told to work on math using an online platform. Students were to complete one math lesson a day. That was it!

As we found out more, I realized that school was going to be closed, at the very least, for three weeks. The second week we were briefed about the many online platforms we would be using, none with which I had any experience. For each new platform, there was daily training that came with a huge learning curve. We would be working through our own learning curve, while teaching our students at the same time.

Suddenly, we now needed to know how to use and navigate Google Meet, Google Classroom, Seesaw, Raz-Kids, Screencastify, Literacy Footprints, Google Chrome, Google Chrome Extensions, Freckle, Epic, Audible, Dreambox, Bridges Math, Google Slides, Google Forms, Google Docs, and Google Sheets. I think I forgot a couple of names.

Teachers not only had to prepare lessons on these platforms, but we also became the computer teacher (IT Director) and troubleshoot students' computer issues. Honestly, I would not have spent the time learning all these platforms without being required to shelter in place. We were instructed that we would also have three Zoom Meetings per week.

My immediate reaction was how do I keep the attention of 24 squirrelly first-graders virtually? Then I thought how do I know that each student is using a device that has access to Zoom? In addition, will they know how to navigate any of the platforms? All of these thoughts swirled in my head as the next problem loomed. How was I going to teach important concepts virtually? Moreover, how will I know my students understand new concepts?

As a first grade teacher, and a year where students are required to learn to read, I wondered how I will be sure that my struggling students will have enough intervention at home to reach the grade-level benchmark. Will the parents know enough to help teach reading? Will there be any way that I can, somehow, teach reading through the computer?

I spent many nights up until 2:00 AM thinking of how this online learning would work and how I could reach my students during this tumultuous time. As a result, I continue to spend approximately 14 hours a day creating and teaching online lessons that I hope will be successful. In addition, teachers also have staff meetings, district grade-level and school grade-level collaboration meetings each week.

Our school grade-level team spends approximately eight hours a week on collaboration, working out ideas and techniques we use for our remote teaching. I continue to fine-tune my lesson plans, to make them easily assessable to students and parents alike. On Zoom, I meet daily with students in small reading groups. Also there are one-on-one Zoom meetings with my four struggling readers. While focusing on the lesson, I try to make Zoom meetings fun. I will tell funny kid jokes, or sing a song, or do a GoNoodle dance while teaching. Encouraging students to be active participants in lessons and sharing what they are learning are important parts of being a first grader.

We do wiggle breaks as needed, go through our days' lesson plans on Seesaw and, at the end, we have a fun scavenger-hunt as their exit ticket. I try to make online learning fun and entertaining while focusing on the skills that need to be learned.

There is another side of teaching with Zoom. There are times where students unmute themselves and you can hear all the noise in their home. I have seen kids jumping on couches, beds, doing TikTok-dances while listening to the lesson, and walking through the house. I have seen and heard siblings argue and some background distractions I'd rather not share.

As a result of teaching online, I have created and implemented an incentive program. I provide positive reinforcement with virtual stickers and virtual rewards. The students earn a point for each assignment turned in, regardless of mistakes, and earn a sticker for every five completed assignments.

A Zoom lunch is offered when a student earns 200 points. Seven of my students have already earned lunch. We eat our lunches together on Zoom and play games like "I Spy" and "20 Questions." We have all loved having this special one-on-one time together!

I honestly was a bit shocked that this idea was so well-received. The rewards of seeing my students smiling faces and of them sharing their homes, toys, and rooms have been wonderful adventures that I would not otherwise have had the opportunity to experience.

What about other areas? Science experiments for my students to try at home are posted on YouTube. Virtual field trips, weekly read-aloud video recordings, daily math lesson videos are also created. We have also had special guests at our meetings such as our Science Specialist, Music Specialist, and Librarian.

I am planning for a virtual talent show for the last week of school. Students will perform their talent virtually for their classmates during our Zoom meeting. With their parent's permission, I will make a personal delivery to each student's home on the last day of school and deliver a gift of masks and gloves. Of course, six foot social distance requirements will be observed.

Through this pandemic, I have learned that I am genuinely appreciated. My students and their parents gave me an incredible parade of cars, parents and kids, signs and decorations galore, celebrating their first grade teacher. Families have sent me gift cards, delivered flowers, wrote sweet messages in chalk in my front yard, sent emails, texts, photographs, pictures, letters, edible bouquets, chocolates, balloons, and most importantly they have imparted their love and support as we travel this journey together.

Teaching is hard, but the benefits far outweigh the challenges. Seeing the light in a child's eyes is worth more than all the money in the world. During this time, my students have expressed to me that they are scared and want to get back to school and normalcy as they once knew it. So do I. I have missed seeing the amazing growth that takes place the last couple of months of school. I will miss celebrating Open House and showcasing student work.

I realized how much I love my job and the importance of interacting with students in the classroom. I know how crucial our role is as their teacher and how I have the ability to impact lives forever. The classroom is a "sanctuary" for learning academically and socially. A school classroom is something that simply cannot be replicated in a virtual classroom.

There is no job I'd rather have then being a teacher of elementary school-age children. I'm pretty sure Covid-19 is an experience that will be etched in these students' minds forever, something never to be forgotten.

I am truly fortunate. I recently was told that I get another year with this same group of students. I am able to "loop" with them and be their second-grade teacher. As we learn together, make up some lost ground, we have the opportunity to continue to touch each other's hearts and lives. As a result of the Covid-19 Pandemic, a bond has been created that will forever link us.

56th Day of Isolation
Anthony Cedoline, PhD

As a psychologist, I spent a career working with adults and children. However, when the Covid-19 virus became a pandemic and shelter-in-place continued for many weeks, I began seeing new kinds of stress and challenges. Here are some of the email comments I have received:

Day 7: Okay, so schools are closed. Do we drop the kids off at the teacher's house?

Day 9: I am homeschooling. The first day I tried to get this kid transferred out of my class.

Day 13: It may take a village to raise a child, but I swear it's going to take a vineyard to homeschool mine.

Day 21: I hope they give us two weeks notice before sending us back out into the real world. I think we'll all need time to become ourselves again. And by "ourselves" I mean lose 10 pounds, cut my hair, and get used to not drinking at 9:00 AM.

Day 30: I am concerned about my new monthly budget: Gas $0, Entertainment $0, Clothes $0, Groceries $2,799.

Day 32: Breaking News: Wearing a mask inside your home is now highly recommended. Not so much to stop Covid-19, but to stop eating."

Day 33: We, low-maintenance women are having our moment right now. We don't have nails to fill and paint, roots to dye, eyebrows to re-ink, and are thrilled not to have to get dressed every day. I have been training for this moment my entire life!

Day 35: When Shelter in Place is over, let's not tell some people.

Day 36: I stepped on my scale this morning. It said: "Please practice social distancing. Only one person at a time on the scale."

Day 39: Appropriate analogy: The curve of new Covid-19 cases is flattening, so we can lift restrictions now. Or could it be said, "The parachute has slowed our rate of descent, so we can take it off now."

Day 40: They say that things may open up soon. I'm staying in until after the second wave of Covid-19 to see what happens to you.

Day 44: People keep asking: "Is coronavirus REALLY that serious?" Listen carefully, the churches and casinos are closed. When heaven and hell agree on the same thing, it's probably pretty serious.

Day 46: Never in a million years could I have imagined I would go up to a bank teller wearing a mask and ask for money.

Day 52: Not to brag, but I haven't been late to anything in almost eight weeks.

Day 54: I was in a long line at 7:45 AM waiting for the grocery store to open at 8:00 AM. Thursday morning is for "seniors only." A young man came from the parking lot and tried to cut in at the front of the line, but an old lady beat him back into the parking lot with her cane.

He returned and tried to cut in again, but an old man punched him in the gut, then kicked him to the ground and rolled him away. Bruised and battered, he approached the line for the third time. He said, “If you people don’t let me unlock the door, none of you will ever get to shop for your groceries.”

Day 56: For the second wave of the Covid-19 pandemic, do we have to stay with the same family or will they relocate me?

These comments resulted in a variety of emotions and they have given me plenty of things to ponder. I know that all of us are truly in this pandemic together. The best way to get to a new normal is to practice the precautions we have been told to practice time and time again. We will overcome Covid-19! What is required is that all of us think of others while we do our part to create the best possible outcome.

COMPASSION, EMPATHY AND HELPING OTHERS

Wash Hands, Wear Masks and Practice Social Distancing!

There appears little doubt that there will be a second wave of Covid-19 and, possibly, a third wave. Historically, the second wave of any pandemic is far worse than the first wave. How big and deadly the second wave of Covid-19 really depends how effectively we all, citizens and government alike, deal with the first wave restrictions. What will people do when we start gathering together again? Will we continue new hygiene habits? Will our economy reopen safely? What happens when millions of people return to work? Will government officials be cautious or over exuberant? Will there be measures available and in place to mitigate a second wave? Will citizens simply fall back into old habits or will families take advantage of what they have learned while sheltering in place. In short, has Covid-19 permanently altered the way many of us think and behave or will we quickly return to the "old" normal? These are all important questions awaiting answers.

Living through the Covid-19 Pandemic has revealed many unexpected results. Many moms and dads are at home. Youngsters are no longer attending school. Members of families are spending far more time together than they ever imagined. Information related to the Pandemic is on the television just about twenty-four hours a day. Sheltering at home has totally changed how many families interact and function.

Hearing stories about how individual families have adapted is fascinating. Across the nation, non-medical people have come up with creative and innovative ideas that help in our fight against Covid-19. In doing so, adults and children have the opportunity to learn about and experience their better selves. The stories in this section share instances of compassion, empathy, and helping others. Perhaps the stories will spark ideas of ways you can help each other get through a second and third wave of Covid-19 and be better for it.

Life Lesson: *The Covid-19 Pandemic has changed our lives. Later in life stories will either be framed as before or after*

Covid-19. There is no doubt that people, including youngsters, will remember the Covid-19 Pandemic for the rest of their lives. As parents we have this time to show our children how we care about other people (people we do not even know), how we show compassion, and how we show others appreciation. To make these lifelong values, we need to have discussions within our families. Even more important, we need to model these values day in and day out for our children. That's the way we create lifelong values and attitudes.

Teenagers Making A Difference

Wash Hands, Wear Masks and Practice Social Distancing!

It should not be surprising how teenagers have taken an active role in helping others during the Covid-19 Pandemic. Often, we adults do not give teens enough credit for their abilities, for their stepping up to help others, and for making a real difference in their communities. Perhaps in our busy lives, we have not taken time to listen, understand, and appreciate them as they move into being adult citizens of our nation. Covid-19 is teaching us a positive lesson about teenagers.

Leave It On The Porch

In a neighborhood where there are a lot of senior citizens live, Kevin and Kavantre, two junior high school boys, came up with a great idea. Since senior citizens citizens are high risk for Covid-19, the boys pick up small items for senior from a nearby open grocery store or pharmacy. The senior citizen calls in an order and pays for it over the phone. One of the boys picks up the order, puts it in a backpack, bikes to the home, and leaves the bag on the front porch of the senior. Each boy tucks a note inside the bag. “We care about you. Stay safe. I am always available to help you. Have a good day.” The boys have found a great way to help others for an hour or two each day.

Let There Be Music

In most communities there are usually a number of good musicians that usually play in the school orchestra or jazz band. Friends in the orchestra and band came up with an idea to support people who are sheltered in place. Helen is quite a violinist and after dinner, she goes around her neighborhood. She stops at each house, rings the door bell and stands well away from the front door, wearing her mask. When the door is answered, Helen plays one or two pieces on her violin.

Robert plays the clarinet in the Jazz Band. The Jazz Band plays a lot of music from the 1930's and 1940's. Robert visits homes where seniors live, rings their door bell, and plays songs from their generation. The smiles on the faces of seniors, as they remember when they were young, is heartwarming.

Anna comes from a large family and plays the guitar. She has learned to play children's songs for her younger brothers and sisters. Now she plays for about an hour in the afternoon, going from door to door playing and singing for young children who are sheltering in place.

Young musicians have considered playing in a trio or quartet. However, social distancing makes playing music together awkward at best, and unsafe at worst. So, let there be music, one musician at a time.

Cutting Up!

Rafael and John have fathers that work in the landscaping business. Each boy has access to a good lawn mower, edger, and burlap tarps. Their idea is to help seniors citizens keep the front lawn of their homes looking nice. They work as a team, mow about ten lawns each Saturday and haul away the grass trimmings. Although the boys accept tips, mowing lawns for seniors is free.

Feed The Undernourished

Churches and community organizations often take on the challenge of providing meals for the poor and homeless. Some programs have existed for many years. Most often feeding programs are staffed by volunteers: retired teachers, nurses, social workers, as well as seniors from all walks of life. Senior citizens have more time to volunteer as well as a lifetime of amazing and helpful experiences. The system has worked well for many years.

Enter Covid-19: One of the group most at risk are senior citizens. Many seniors felt they could no longer come in contact with people who could, evenly remotely, have Covid-19. In addition, organizations feeding the homeless could no longer serve meals inside buildings.

What to do? Hungry people still need to be fed.

- Move feeding programs outside.
- Recruit volunteer teenagers to be in charge of the outside distribution of meals.
- Volunteer seniors prepare sack breakfasts and lunches in organizational kitchens the day before they are needed. Sack meals are stored in refrigerators.
- Completely sanitize tables before and after serving food.
- Set up tables outside with sack meals.

- Mark sidewalks to help people maintain proper social distance.
- Volunteers always wear masks!

STAR
ROOM
— SERVING THOSE AROUND US —
Matthew 25: 35 NLV
"For I was hungry and you gave Me food to eat. I was
gave Me water to drink. I was a stranger and you gave Me
Guests are welcome to come to our
STAR Room for Food, shelter + comfort ~
First Baptist

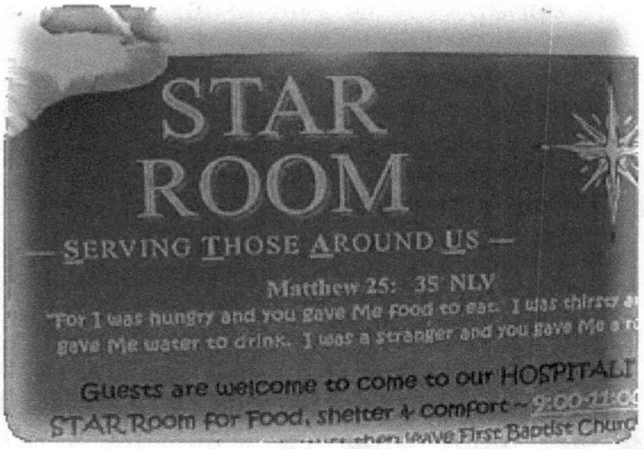

A young friend named Liam told me, "The need to keep feeding the poor and homeless is how my mother and I came involved in the STAR Program. As a junior high student, I like helping people who need food and they really like me."

Story Time

Suzie and Maria both have younger sisters and brothers that love to have stories read to them. Both use their voices very well and add body movements when they read a book. Suzie and Maria have teamed up and read two stories over the computer just about the time most toddlers take a nap. Shelter in place moms love the idea that someone else is entertaining their young children, at least for a few minutes.

Appreciation Signs

A group of high school art students obtained poster boards to make "thank you" or "appreciation" signs. They contacted senior citizens and offered to make them a sign of their choice to put it in their front window. The seniors now have a way of giving thanks publically and the art students did a project that made a difference for the elderly in their community.

Another group cut poster boards in half and delivered them to families with kids who are sheltering in place. Family members work together to create a "thank you" sign for their front window.

Contacting people they do not know is always a problem for teens. However, teens are good problem solvers. They start by asking mom or dad to help with people they know. Members of clubs, volunteer organizations, and churches often have rosters. It does not take many adults to help get things going.

Dog Walking

Whether we are in a pandemic or not, dogs still need to be walked. Elderly people are at a high risk for contracting Covid-19 and, as a result, often elect not to leave their homes. A teen can be a welcome solution that is a genuine help to both dogs and owners. There are a few basic rules:

- Dogs must always be on a leash.
- Carry and know how to use "poop" bags.
- Stay clear of other dogs and people.

- Always wear a face mask.
- Thirty minutes is enough time for a good walk (Always check with the owner for the length of a walk.)

Walking a dog is not only good for the dog, it also helps teens burn off extra energy.

Helping Younger Siblings

In certain subject areas, we parents may feel hopelessly out of date. Enlisting the help of an older teen to help a younger sibling may be one answer. Depending on the teen and the relationship between the teen and younger child, approaching this kind of request may be tricky.

"We are in this together." is a phase we have all heard. We all have to support each other to get through this pandemic, is a reality. Simply stating the concern about the difficulty a younger sibling is having in a subject opens the way for an honest two-way discussion with an older teen about the possibility of helping. If the teen is willing, agree on certain parameters: subject, length of time each day, and approach. There are three basic principles that help the teen maximizes feeling of success.

- Model – In simple terms, the teen explains and demonstrates the skill or concept. Sometimes it takes several approaches, using different words, before the youngster begins to understand.
- Lead – Together walk through each step... do it together. Sometimes, this takes more than one try.
- Test – The youngster does it on his/her own.

- Praise – "Good job." "You are getting it." "I can see the effort you are making."

Limiting the time is important. Twenty to thirty minutes of helping a younger sibling is usually "enough for each of them."

Following a Dream

Many teens develop special interests, something they feel passionate about, want to know a lot about or something that may lead to a career. Some of the time spent sheltering in place can be used to explore a dream, dig deeper into it, learn how it relates to other areas in their life.

Years ago, I remember a lot of youngsters wanting to be a pilot. Being a pilot was the only job in flying they knew about. Other than being a flight attendant, they had no idea of other related jobs: ground crew, jet engine mechanic, ticket agent, aircraft controller, baggage handler, and on and on. Fortunately today, teens can do a lot of exploring through the use of technology.

Teens having a passion may not lead to a career. However, learning more gives them a much broader understanding of career possibilities. For some, maybe that dream will inspire them for a lifetime.

Repurposing Political Signs

Wash Hands, Wear Masks and Practice Social Distancing!

A group of middle school friends spent a lot of time talking to each other on the phone and playing games during sheltering in place. One of the moms said to her daughter, "Why don't your friends do something positive instead of sitting around and yakking for hours on the phone? The daughter did not take the comment well, but her friend on the other end did and came up with an idea. Their state had just had a primary election and there were campaign signs everywhere. The seven friends used "Zoom" to have a planning session.

The next morning each girl and boy in the group put on a face mask. Each one, individually, went around their neighborhood collecting as many old political signs as possible (In this state, election signs have to be removed within a week anyway). When the friends checked in, they had collected thirty-four signs. Step one of the plan was successful.

The next challenge was to find white paper to cover the signs. So many stores were closed, sheets of white paper were hard to come by. They told their mothers about their plan and enlisted moms to try and get butcher paper when they went to the grocery store. When the butchers learned of the plan, they gladly donated several feet of butcher paper. Step two of the plan was successful.

The group wanted the lettering to be brightly colored so messages could easily be seen. Group members shared ideas of where to find paint. Craft stores, they thought were sources for paint, were closed. Paint was available at big hardware stores, but who needs a gallon of paint for thirty-four signs? Finding paint, much less bright colors that would stand out, was not as easy as they thought. One of the dads overheard the discussion. He suggested they ask their dads if they had any partial cans of old paint in the garage. Almost everyone had old cans of paint and a variety of colors too. Step three of the plan was successful.

WE LOVE
NURSES
THANK YOU
THANK YOU
HEALTH
CARE
WORKERS
THANK YOU
EMT'S
AND
THANK YOU
AMBULANCE
DRIVERS
THANK YOU
HOSPITAL
CLEANING
STAFF
THANK YOU
DAY CARE
PROVIDERS
FOR TAKING CARE
OF
FIRST RESPONDER'S
CHILDREN
THANK YOU
TEACHERS
FOR
ONLINE LESSONS
THANK YOU
FRIENDS FOR
SUPPORTING
FIRST
RESPONDERS
THANK YOU
SUPER MARKET CLERKS
FOR KEEPING FOOD
ON THE SHELVES
THANK YOU
ESSENTIAL WORKERS
YOU DO SO MUCH THAT WE
DON'T THINK ABOUT

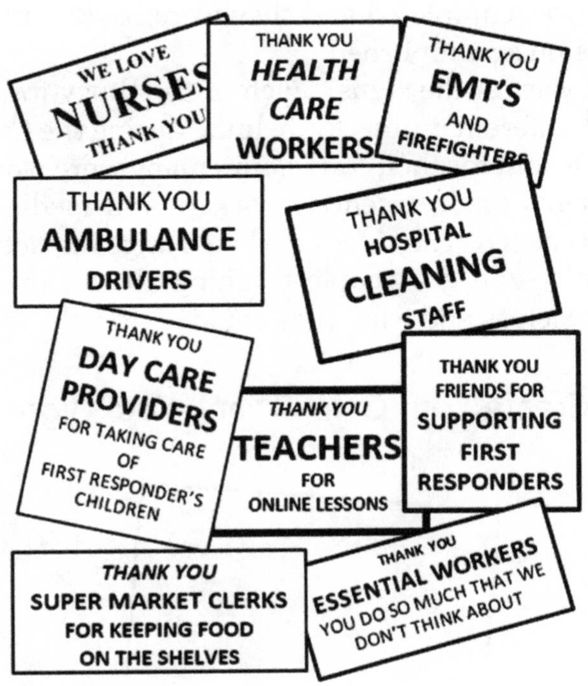

On their next "Zoom" call, they spend an hour discussing what should be painted on each sign. Then each member spent the day painting words on their signs and outlining each letter with a contrasting color. Creating the signs was more work than they imagined. Step four of the plan was successful.

That evening, the group discussed where to put the signs and how to coordinate time so that all the signs were placed within an hour or two. Step five of the plan was agreed upon.

Early the next morning, precisely at 7:00 AM, each member put on their protective face mask, gathered their signs, and headed down the streets. Most of the signs ended up streets that are well traveled. By 7:45 AM, their mission was completed and they were back home. Step six: Mission accomplished!

What was on the signs? Each of the thirty four signs thanked different groups for helping during the Covid-19 Pandemic and for their long hours many were working.

The signs made essential workers and medical staff feel appreciated. The signs also had a huge impact on the community and got people thinking about others, not just themselves and what they could do to help.

Create Your Own "Thank You" Sign

Face Mask Shortages

Wash Hands, Wear Masks and Practice Social Distancing!

Most people know there has been a real shortage of face masks during the Covid-19 Pandemic. In many towns, individual and small groups of teens banded together to help fill the need for face masks. Teens get very creative in both maintaining social distance and wearing protective face masks. When Junior High Schools and High Schools reopen, there will be a ready- made market for handmade "designer" face masks. Selling masks can become quite a fundraiser for a school club or community organization.

There were individual teens sewing at home and making a few of dozen masks each week to meet a specific need for a small number of masks:

- Masks for the homeless.
- Masks for volunteers who provide breakfast, lunch, or dinner for the homeless
- Masks for volunteers helping non-profit organizations.
- Masks for bus drivers.
- Masks for local gas station employees
- Masks for low income families who may not be able to afford store bought masks.
- Masks for public service groups: police, fire, paramedics, postmen, etc.

The pandemic helped individual teens realize they have skills they can use to help others and make a difference.

In larger towns and small cities, groups of teens banded together to sew large numbers of masks. Group members wore distinctive masks when they worked together sewing masks for others. They also set aside work areas that allowed for proper social distancing.

- A small group of teens gathered little-used sewing machines and set up a sewing shop in a garage. The group literally produced hundreds of masks each week.
- Some owners of fabric stores created partnerships by providing fabric remnants and elastic materials to small groups of teen mask makers.
- The idea of "designer" masks became a fad in some areas. Teens sell designer masks at a low price and use the profits to buy materials and create masks that were donated to homeless shelters, assisted living homes, and other organizations where masks are in short supply.
- One high school group and an owner of a silk screen shop teamed up to make masks imprinted with their high school mascot.
- Another group made masks with their local professional sports team logos on them.
- A group of Jewish teens made masks out of old yarmulkes, a coffee filter, and wide rubber bands. The masks were give to Jewish homes for the aged.

Teenagers are realizing they can make a big impact when they join together and use their talent and energy in a common cause for good. Of course, all these teen groups know the importance of practicing social distancing and wearing masks.

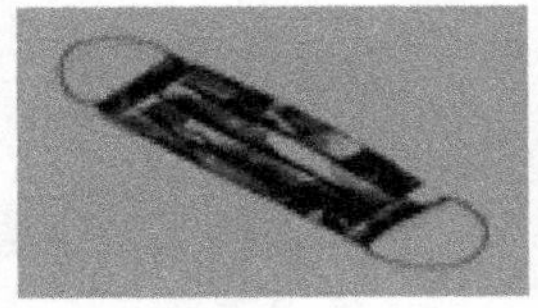 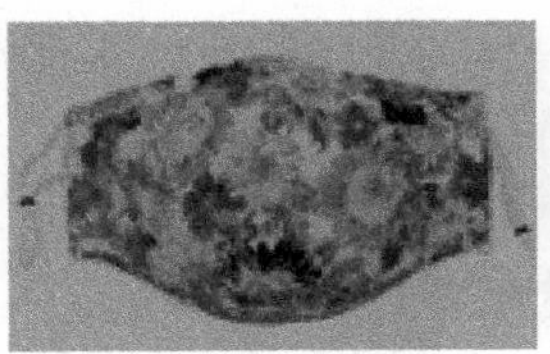 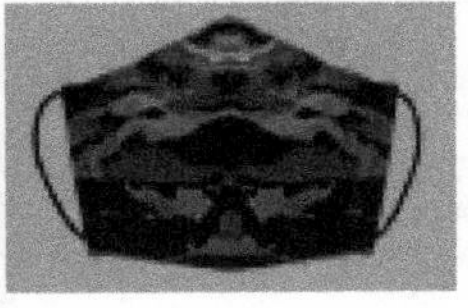

What do these examples mean? They mean that teens have more ideas, energy, and empathy than most people could ever imagine. Covid-19 has provided teens an opportunity to share their compassion for others and make a real difference in showing appreciation for medical workers who are involved with helping the victims of Covid-19 and essential workers who do so much in helping each of us stay safe.

Life Lesson: *Teens have a lot more talent and ability than most of us give them credit for. Yes, these are unusual times that will affect how we think for the rest of our lives. Perhaps we will use this experience to change the way we think as well as believe that teens have the ability to make a difference and the world a little bit better.*

YOUNGER AGE CHILDREN

Wash Hands, Wear Masks and Practice Social Distancing!

Shelter in Place with younger children is a mixed bag. On one hand, they require more direct supervision, have a smaller attention span, and can get "whiney." Just ask any mom. On the other hand, they can be sweet, lovable, and helpful.

Most younger children have a lot of energy, need to change activities more often, and require more adult guidance: school work, play time, getting along with siblings, and helping around the house. Taking time to talk and plan with them each day can be a great help. So is having a written schedule/chart with spaces to fill in particular times and things to do each day. Think about how their day is scheduled at school and try to mirror it.

Appropriately involving younger children in decision making can create buy-in, a sense of responsibility and new a habit. Would you rather start school work at 8:30 AM or 9:00 AM?

Would you rather set the table for breakfast or put the dishes in the sink after we eat?

When you have a break, what game would you like to play in the back yard?

Television is not on during the day at school. The same should be true at home.

Hand Washing

(Sing to the melody of "This Is the Way We Brush Our Teeth")

This is the way we wash our hands, wash our hands, wash our hands.
This is the way we wash our hands, many times a day.
This is the way we wash our fingers, wash our fingers, wash our fingers.
This is the way we wash our fingers, many times a day.
This is the way we wash our thumbs, wash our thumbs, wash our thumbs.
This is the way we wash our thumbs, many times a day.
This is the way we scrub our nails, scrub our nails, scrub our nails.
This is the way we scrub our nails, many times a day.
Now my hands are good and clean, good and clean, good and clean.
I am keeping Covid-19 far, far away.

Life Lesson: *Helping youngsters, especially the very young, learn the important of good hygiene, including washing hands completely during the pandemic, can become good lifelong habits. There is no better time to start than when there is an obvious need.*

Mathematics At Home

Whether it is distance learning or packets sent home, most schools provide specific assignments for children during these pandemic times when schools are closed.

When your child is learning a mathematical skill or operation, it is helpful for an adult or teenager to be there. Sometimes the person answers questions or explain things using different words. If the child is having difficulty completing an assignment, try to come up with a different way or example to explain what the child needs to know. Older children can also help younger siblings make flash cards.

Shelter at home provides a lot of opportunities for a child to learn about the practical side of mathematics, how mathematics is used every day in real life situations. Some activities around the house might include youngsters walking around the house and making a list of everything that is a rectangle. Another time they can make list of circles, squares, arcs, triangle. Similar activities can be done outside. These are good ways to help youngsters see how math and geometry are a part of everyday life . Another activity is to have a discussion on what kind of jobs require a knowledge of mathematics.

- How do doctors use math?
- How do carpenters use math?
- How do computers use math?
- How do cooks and bakers use math?

Mathematics And Cooking

Many families have a children's cook book tucked away somewhere. I still do not know where ours is, but I have seen it in the past when grandchildren visit and are excited to make something with Grandma.

Parents are often just plain too busy to spend the time helping their children learn how to cook. It's a great time to find out why they like certain foods and what kinds of foods you ate as a child. Sheltering at Home provides a unique opportunity for child parent time in the kitchen.

- Do some simple cooking together. Just learning the basics of preparing a meal is a good thing.
- Mathematics can be easily included if you use a cookbook. A child's cookbook is a great way to start learning...a cup of (8oz), two tablespoons of, how many teaspoons are in a tablespoon, how many cookies will this recipe make? How many cookies are in a dozen? When cooking pasta, what size pot is recommended and how much water should be in the pot? You'll come up with even better ideas.
- A ruler or tape measure is another way to help youngstsers understand how we use mathematics in our everyday lives. Some examples might include measuring the depth of a kitchen shelf. Will dinner plates fit on the shelf? Is there any extra space? Measure the height of the kitchen table and the counter top. If they are different, why?

What is the width of various doors. Why might some be different? Older kids can use a tape measure to find out the area of a drawer, etc. Why are some drawers larger or smaller or are deeper?

- How many gallons will the kitchen sink hold, the bathroom sink?
- Choosing one different practical math activity each day, can create a real understanding of how math is used in our everyday life.

Journaling

Journaling is something that youngsters of all ages can do. The Covid-19 is a stressful time for everyone, including children. It's hard for all of us to see unexpected changes happening in our lives...especially changes that affect everyone around us. Journaling is a good way to put stress into words as well as give children a way to express how they are feeling each day about what is happening around them.

- Younger children draw a picture of something that happened each day. Date each picture and have your child tell you about their picture. You might want to write one or two sentences at the bottom. Clip them together to share later.
- Grades 1-3 can draw a picture on the top half of a page and write from one sentence to a three or four sentence paragraph. The

following is one way of helping a youngster develop a paragraph.

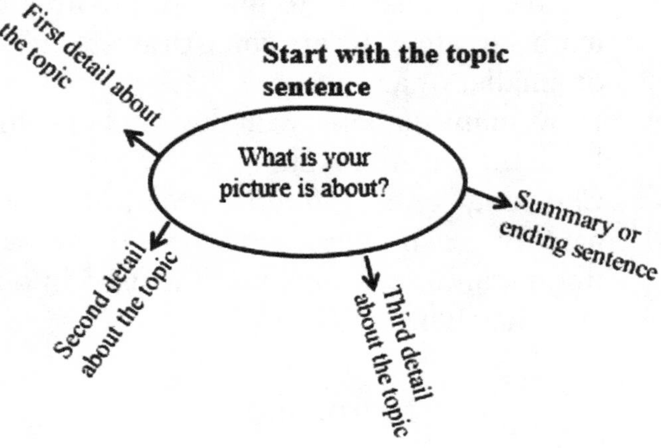

Drawing and writing are good ways for youngster to express how they are feeling...especially in a time of stress. Parents can also ask simple questions to help kids open up and how they may be feeling.

- Can you tell me more about this idea or this part of a picture?
- What part of the picture do you like best?
- This is an interesting word. Can you tell me more about what you were thinking?

Again, date and clip each story together so they can be shared later...especially when they become adults!

Hand Print Note Cards

Another great project for younger children is making "hand print" cards using tempera or other water soluble paint. Brush a little bit of paint on their hands at a time. Kids tend to want to stick their whole hand in paint. Try handprints out on a piece of newspaper or other scrap paper until they get idea and find a "look" they like. The same idea can be used to make wrapping paper.

Writing Appreciation Notes

Many younger children know the name of someone who is really important to them. Children can certainly write a paragraph to tell these people how much they are appreciated. After the first letter or two, children can begin to write patients with Covid-19 and to medical people working in the hospital.

Get Well Cards

Being in the hospital or a nursing home is bad enough, but when family members cannot visit it is ten times worse. Young children can bring a smile to a face of a senior citizen when they open a get well or greeting card from an elementary school age youngsters.

Four to six cards can be made by four to six year old children over a few days. The art work is uplifting and a few words about getting well are enough. Second through fifth graders can write a message or make up a poem.

A parent can make a phone call to find out how to address a large envelope, containing all the cards, so they will get to the patients.

Rainbow On The Window

Rainbows are a traditional symbol of better times ahead. Young children can create a rainbow picture and put it on the front window. They can also make a rainbow get well card. A bit of science can also be taught. A rainbow is simply light broken into component colors through raindrops or a prism. The colors in a rainbow are always arranged the same: red, orange, yellow, green, blue, indigo, and violet.

Sock Puppets

Most of us have a one-of-a-kind socks in the back of a drawer or box. Making sock puppets, using a variety of different socks, is a great activity. Socks can be decorated with felt tip pens, buttons, etc. Since there are various sizes of socks in most homes, a sock family can be created. Everyone in the family can have a different sock puppet and make up stories or a plays together.

Collages

Old magazines are a great source for creating a collage. Topics could be animals, trees, sports, toys, of anything that interests a child. Going through magazines and cutting out pictures can take a good amount of time and putting a collage together with paste or glue can take even more time.

Another kind of collage can be made from plastic milk jugs. With a bit of help and guidance, a plastic milk jug can be cut out into the shapes of various animals: pigs, elephant, bear, dog, etc. Cutting out shapes of colored paper and gluing them on the milk carton gives texture as does adding things such as pipe cleaners. This project does require some discussion about animals, shapes, and how to cut out legs and other parts. Working with a plastic milk jug is good project for a dad and child working together as a team.

A Back Yard Par Course

Liam's and Izzy's mom made a par course in the back yard. The boys run, jump, balance, serpentine, as well as do sit-ups, jumping jacks, waist twists, bouncing a ball the same number of times as their age, and making one last shot into a bucket. (The ball in the bucket leaves the activity ready for the next person.) After an hour of school work, spending fifteen minutes on the obstacle course can be a welcome break.

Hopscotch

Using sidewalk chalk, it's easy to make an old fashion hopscotch game on a walkway or patio. Hopscotch is a great game to develop balance and bending skills. It's also a game that siblings can play together.

Jump Rope

Jump Rope is another traditional game. If you have several children, the older ones can teach younger ones how to jump rope. Jump rope is a great way to develop coordination skills.

Making An Inside "Hideout"

As kids, many of us made a tent inside the house. Sheltering in Place is an opportunity to expand on the idea. Use an old sheet (the bigger, the better) as the covering for the tent. Work in a place where crayons, felt tip markers, colored pens, etc. will not transfer onto carpets or floors such as a patio or garage floor. If you have several children, divide the tent into sections for each youngster. It may take a couple days do the actual art work. Set up the hideout using chairs, tables, or other items around the house as a frame.

Play-Doh

If you do not already have play-doh at home, there are several easy recipes online. Adding a drop or two of food coloring and letting kids kneed and store play-doh in small containers with lids. It's a great way to have an extra activity tucked away just in case you need one.

River Rock Paper Weights

Smooth river rock about the size of a youngster's hand make a great paper weight gift. Painting an animal, flower, or name is a good activity requiring the use of small hand muscles. There may be a few leftover pieces of tile in the garage that makes a great base when the rock is glued on.

Cardboard Box Apartments

Two brothers found old cardboard boxes. Most boxes were small to medium size, but there were a few big ones. Then the boys spent a couple of days taping boxes closed so they were sturdy. They cut connecting holes in boxes so they could crawl from one box to another. The big boxes became place for the boys to hang out and play with toys or legos. Smaller boxes were decorated and stacked on each other. The smaller boxes became upper floor apartments. The cat picked out a high box apartment for his own space. Everyone laughed when they saw the cat climb up the side and into his apartment for some peace and quiet.

Treasure Hunt

If there are two or three children sheltering in place together, a treasure hunt is a good bonding activity. Each child picks out ten small objects or toys. One of the other children hides the items on the patio or small back yard. When one child is trying to find his/her items, the others cheer him on. The next child's items are then hidden and found.

A modification of the treasure hunt is to time the hunt to find out who find the items that fastest. If an item is not found, all the players look. There are lots of possible versions of a treasure hunt. Kids can even make up treasure hunts for the parents.

The Alphabet Game

The alphabet is a simple game that helps young children think of words by categories. It can also be played by a team of a younger and older child, or by two teams of a parent and child.

ALPHABET GAME

	Name	***Food***	***Toy***
A	Angie	apple	airplane
B	Ben	berries	boat
C	Carrie	carrots	car
D	Danna	dates	
E	Emmy	endive lettuce	
F	Francisco	French fries	
G	Geri		
H	Henry		
I	Izzy		
J	Juanita		
K	Kerry		
L	Lucy		
M			
etc.			

Vegetable Garden

A vegetable garden can be a small plot of land next to a fence, several larger flower pots, or even a larger area in the backyard. All these areas can be used to grow vegetables. A vegetable garden can be a family affair or each youngsters is assigned a small area or a couple of containers.

Find out which vegetables are easy to grow in your area and the time of year they should be planted. Preparing the soil...hoeing weeds, turning the soil using a shovel, making sure the soil is loose and not packed, making furrows, are just some ways of getting the soil ready for seeds. Be sure the youngstsers read and follow the directions on the package. Finally, create a log from planting to harvest.

Sample Garden Log

Activity	Date	Seeds	Plants	Height
Prepare soil	5-25			
Plant	5-27	Bean Seeds	Tomato Plants	3" high
Schedule	5-28			
Watering	6-13	First sprout	Tomato Plants	5" high
Every other	6-20	1 " high		
Day	6-30	3 " high	Tomato flowers	7" high
	7-15	Flowers	Sm. Tomatoes	8" high
	-----		First Harvest	

When youngsters actually grow vegetables and prepare them, they are far more likely to eat them...even ones they may not like.

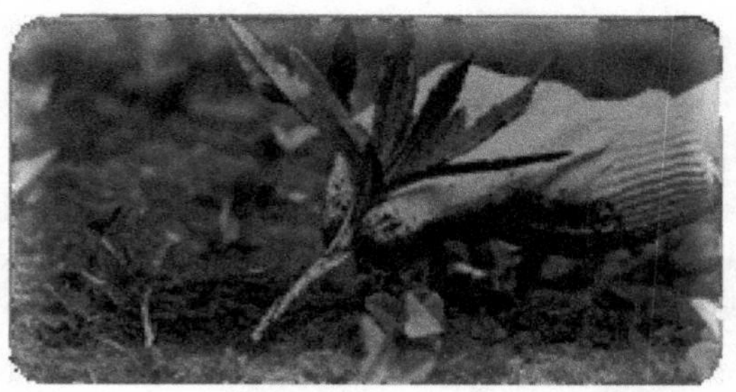

Weed Pulling Contest

Having three children at home 24/7 is a "stretch" for any parent. Working together, children and parents, can create new activities and ones that can be a challenge.

About six week into Shelter In Place, one mom, with three young kids, was ready to start "pulling out her hair." Her frustration gave her an idea...pulling out the weeds. The ground was fairly soft due to some recent rains and the time was right. Here are the rules of the contest.

- The contest lasts for only 15 minutes.
- Each child gets a box for the weeds they pick.
- To count, the weed must have the root attached.
- Size does not count...only weeds with roots count.
- Each child counts the weeds in front of mom and the siblings.
- The winner gets to choose the family game for the evening. (I am sure you can come up with other prizes.)

The game worked. Mom got away with the kids playing the game about three times. Then the kids caught on. All good ideas come to an end. I am sure you can come up with equally good ideas...just do not pull out your hair.

Daddy Led Activities

Wooden Toys

Some dads have shops in the garage, others may have a handsaw, a drill and sandpaper. Most dads have a few pieces of scrap wood. With a little imagination, youngsters can make their own wooden toys. Toy kits can also be ordered online.

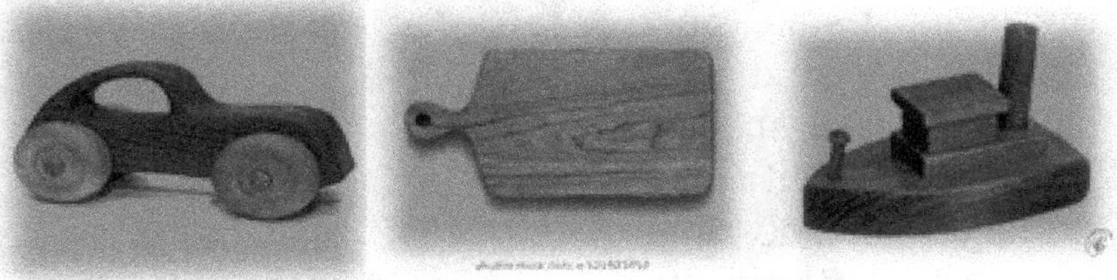

The three items above are samples of hundreds of toy kits that are available on line if dad is not into woodworking. When I made toys with my grandchildren, we always signed the bottom with our names and the date. Twenty years later, the grandkids still have their toys that show a lot of wear and tear.

Night Out

Night out is not a night out with the "Boys." Rather it is a night out with your kids. If you have a tent, great! If not, a couple of large blankets over two ropes work just as well. If you have a tarp of some kind it helps keep the night moisture away. Sleeping bags or heavy blankets both work for sleeping...if you have air mattresses, even better. Flashlights of any kind are a must.

A BBQ with hamburgers, hot dogs, and grilled vegetables make a great dinner for the campers. An outside dinner also gives dad the opportunity to cook with the kids.

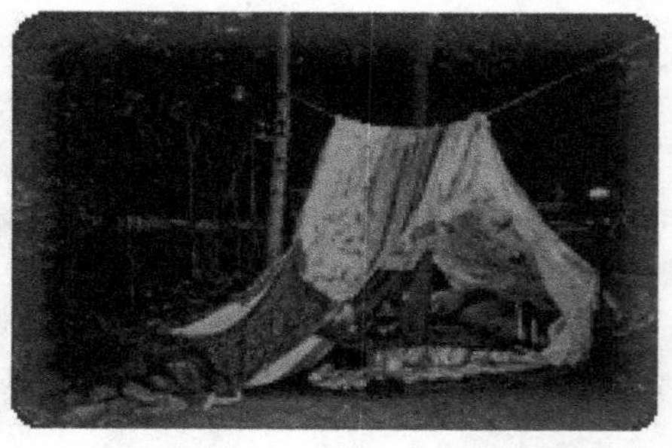

When it is time to go inside the tent, a whole new adventure can begin. Using your fingers, you and the kids can make shapes like animals. With the flashlight on one side of your hand, the shape will a shadow on the side of the tent. Another activity is to create a round robin story. Dad starts a story, followed by each person adding to the story as each person take turns. Funny stories and ghost stories both work well. In addition, games like checkers, Uno, Sorry or a favorite game can be played before bedtime.

Dad "camping" with the kids will create a long lasting memory. "Dad, remember when we..."

Losing At games

Children love playing games, especially seeing "Dad Lose." Whether it is a game like checkers, Uno, or Fish, kids love seeing a parent make a "big" mistake or losing. It is even more fun when the act of losing is animated.

"Oh no! Did I really do that?"

SMALL BUSINESSES

Wash Hands, Wear Masks and Practice Social Distancing!

Almost all people have taken the Covid-19 Pandemic and restrictions from their governors very seriously. Sheltering in place, wearing face masks, and practicing good hygiene are now part of everyday life. Almost all businesses closed and waited until being told they could begin the reopening process. Some small business use telephones, computers, and home delivery to serve customer needs. Other small businesses, often restaurants, have developed take out systems. Most owners of small business are struggling to survive. However, more and more are coming up with creative ways to help bridge the Covid-19 closure gap.

Feeding Hospital Workers

In large industrial areas there are often restaurants that thrive by providing breakfast and lunch to hungry workers. Some restaurants actually serve hundreds of meals a day and go through tremendous amounts of food. Restaurants usually order food from wholesalers twice a week.

One such restaurant had just received a large food order. The next day it was ordered to close as a result of the rapidly spreading Covid-19 pandemic. The storage shelves were full. The cold storage unit was full. The freezer was full.

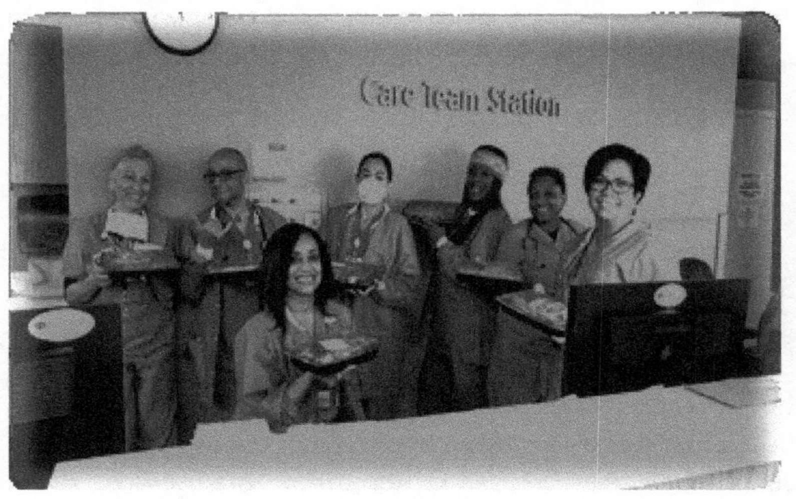

As the restaurant owner watched the havoc the Covid-19 virus was having on his community and the health care system. He was in awe of something that been beyond comprehension just a few days before. He saw pictures of health workers on television that looked completely exhausted from helping very ill patients and how they were reacting as the number of patients dying increased at an alarming rate. A friend was hospitalized with the Covid-19 virus. He had to do something to help!

Realizing that his restaurant was fully stocked with food, the restaurant owner contacted the hospital. Quickly, a plan was created to serve free hot meals to over a hundred hospital workers two shifts a day...

doctors, nurses, paraprofessionals, laundry staff, and cleaning staff...until the restaurant ran out of food. Four restaurant employees were brought back to work.

However, the food did not run out. Once the local television station heard about the free meals for health care workers they aired the story. For months, additional food stocks and money have been provided by individual donations and wholesale businesses. The hot food project for hospital workers continues.

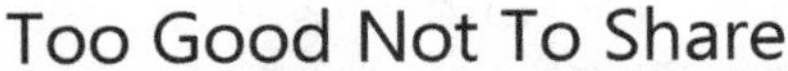

Too Good Not To Share

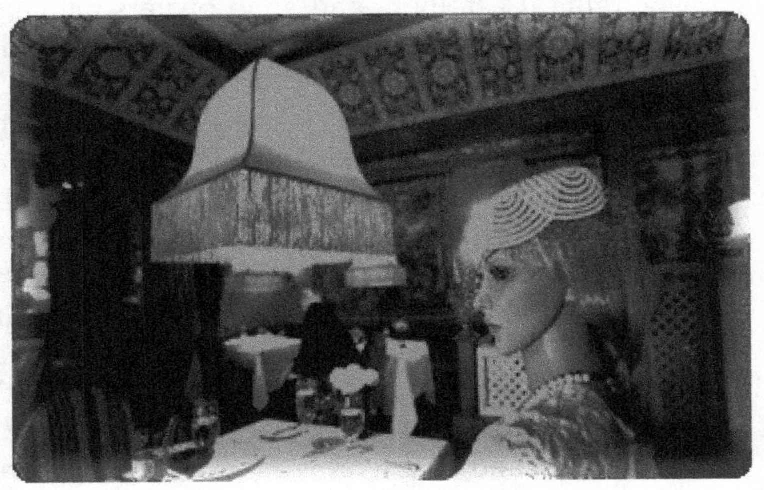

The Inn at Little Washington, a famous three-star Michelin restaurant in Virginia, approached reopening for inside dining in a wonderfully unique way. Their idea may spark hundreds of other ideas around the nation that may help restaurants financially survive during the lengthy Covid-19 Pandemic.

The Inn at Little Washington created a way to help diners abide by the social distancing guidelines while enjoying dinner in a unique environment. Diners are seated next to completely set tables with beautifully 1940's style dressed mannequins.

Chef Patrick O'Connell said. "This would allows plenty of space between guests and elicits a few smiles and provides some fun photo ops."

1882 Grille

A small city prides itself on its beautiful tree-lined vintage main street and its wide variety of local shops and restaurants. Customers and shop owners actually know each other. Residents take pride in that fact that no chain stores are allowed in the downtown area.

The 1882 Grill is a popular family restaurant on the second floor of a quaint old building. Its location requires most customers to use an elevator. The food is excellent, the prices are reasonable, and the view of the surrounding downtown area is spectacular. Like most restaurants, Covid-19 forced the 1882 Grille to shut their doors. Only a few restaurants were easily adapted to a "Take Out Only" situation. However, doing "take out" from the second floor? You have got to be kidding!

As government and health officials thought they were getting a handle on Covid-19, discussions were started about how to do a careful, one small step at a time, reopening of some businesses. Some shops were open to one customer at a time. A customer waited outside the door wearing a mask and gloves. Social distancing lines were marked on the sidewalks. When one person left the store, another person is allowed to go in. The process worked well. However, it did not seem viable for a restaurant on a second floor.

Finally, a plan was formed to reopen 1882 Grille... DRIVE BY! The staff selected a few entrees from the menu that could be adapted to take out. The 1882 Grille used Facebook to contact as many customers as possible. Customers could call in orders for two or three of the entrees and pick them up between 4 PM and 6:30

PM for their reopening. Dinners were free on opening day. Community response to the reopening the 1882 Grille was beyond anyone's imagination

On, Saturday, six long folding tables were put at the curb of the street. 7500 meals were nicely packaged and put into labeled paper bags. Bags were brought down the elevator to the tables. About 2000 bags sat on curbside tables waiting to be picked up.

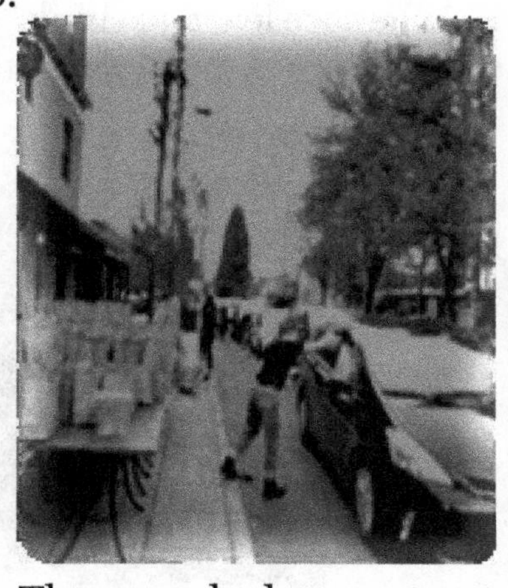

Restaurant staff greeted people in each car, checked their order. Of course, everyone was wearing brightly colored masks. Firefighters and restaurant staff put dinner bags into each car through the passenger side window. There were so many cars that members of the police department directed traffic. They marked one street for driving to the restaurant, closed a side street for the actual pickup, and then directed traffic when and how to turn onto the main street of town to leave.

When a whole town decides a community business is really worth saving, amazing things actually happen!

The 1882 Grille is now back in business, taking phone orders, cooking, and selling DRIVE BY lunches and dinners each day.

Incahoots

Incahoots is popular little shop where you can sit and have tea and shortbread, buy a beautiful bouquet of flowers, or shop for gifts and garden plants. Covid-19 shut them down immediately. No customers, no tea, no income!

Incahoots is noted for creativity. On the parking lot side of the building there is a storeroom with a fairly large window. Idea! Take everything out of the storeroom. Install a counter outside the window. Create a drive-through. Incahoots is open for drive-through business including tea and shortbread.

When we learn to think "out of the box," new solutions often happen...even in a storeroom. Way to go!

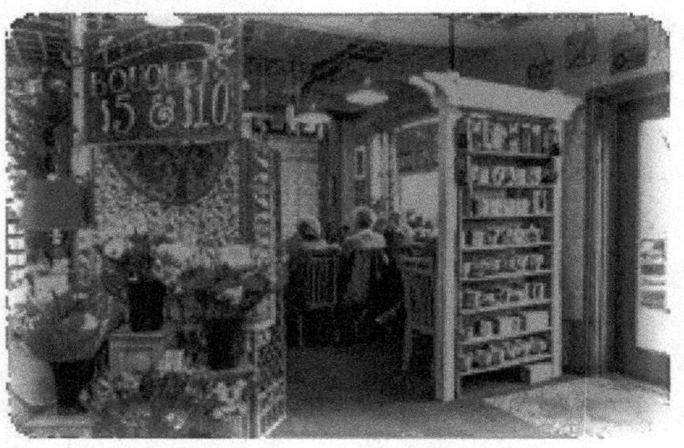

Hopscotch Toy Store

Kids, parents, and grandparents love Hopscotch Toy Store. It's a locally-owned shop that really focuses on kids. The mix of toys and games caters to a wide variety of ages and interests. When a youngster is going to have a birthday party, Hopscotch will help the child put together a basket of party prizes.

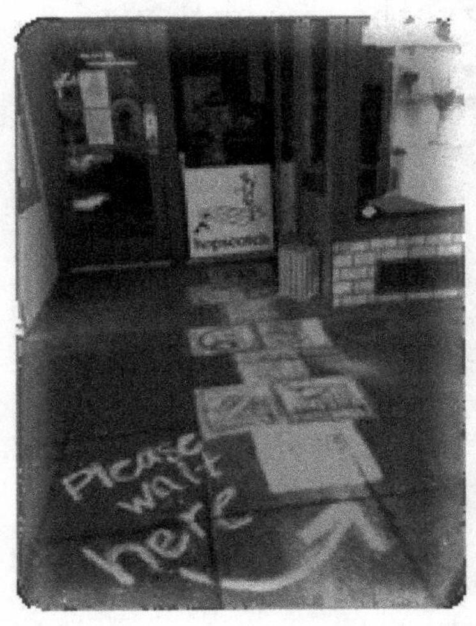

Naturally, as a result of the Covid-19 Pandemic, Hopscotch was closed. The business has survived because of phone orders and delivery service. With the partial lifting of restrictions, Hopscotch has reopened as a "take out." Hopscotch is located in an old building on the main downtown street.

It has two doors. One door remains locked. The other door is open and the owner has put a large desk across it. While wearing masks, customers can walk up to the desk. While social distancing, toys can be purchased or picked up.

If it is the day of a birthday, the child and his mother are allowed to come inside the story to pick out toys. Of course masks and social distancing are required. Izzy was celebrating his sixth birthday. His excited comment to his mom was, "Do we really get to go inside Hopscotch because it's my birthday? Yippee!"

Dining In: Different Approach

Despite financial help from the Federal Government, there remains concern that hundreds of thousands of restaurants across the country will not survive the economic ravages of the Covid-19 Pandemic. Even if allowed to reopen, there will be restrictions on the number of customers allowed. One estimate is that many restaurants may end up with a new capacity of only twenty-five percent...which may not be enough to survive.

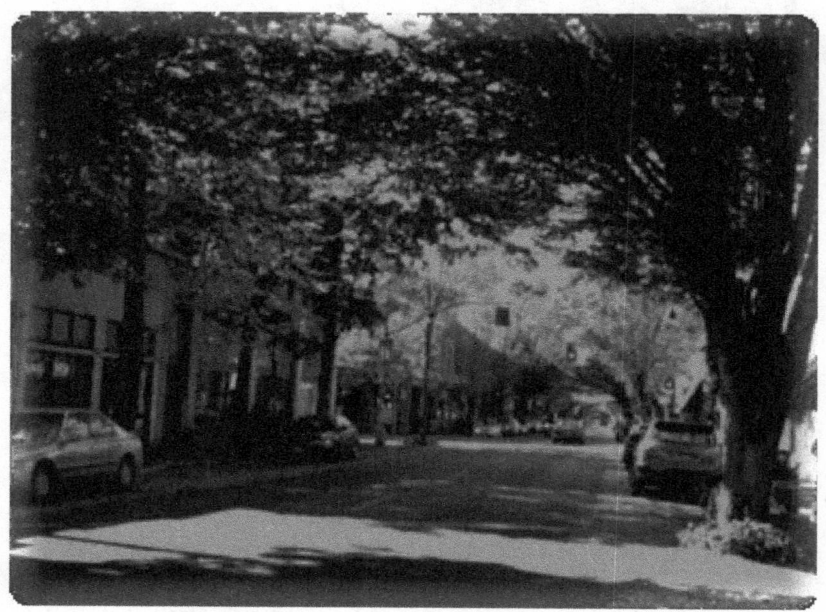

This small Oregon city has a wonderful downtown street that is reserved for only small, independent businesses. Chain stores are all located away from downtown. Except for a few restaurants which offered take-out, Covid-19 shut down the entire street.

As restrictions begin to relax, some business people are having discussions about actually closing the main street each weekend and making it into an outdoor "eating mall". The concept would allow the many restaurants to expand their capacity out onto the actual street and dramatically increase business while creating "social distance" between tables.

In other small cities, where street malls are permanent, different kinds of planters and other unique barriers have added to create a wonderful outdoor dining experience. Because of many people dining on the main street, other types of business greatly benefited from the relaxed atmosphere and additional foot traffic.

The question is, "Will this beautiful small city in Oregon actually make it happen?"

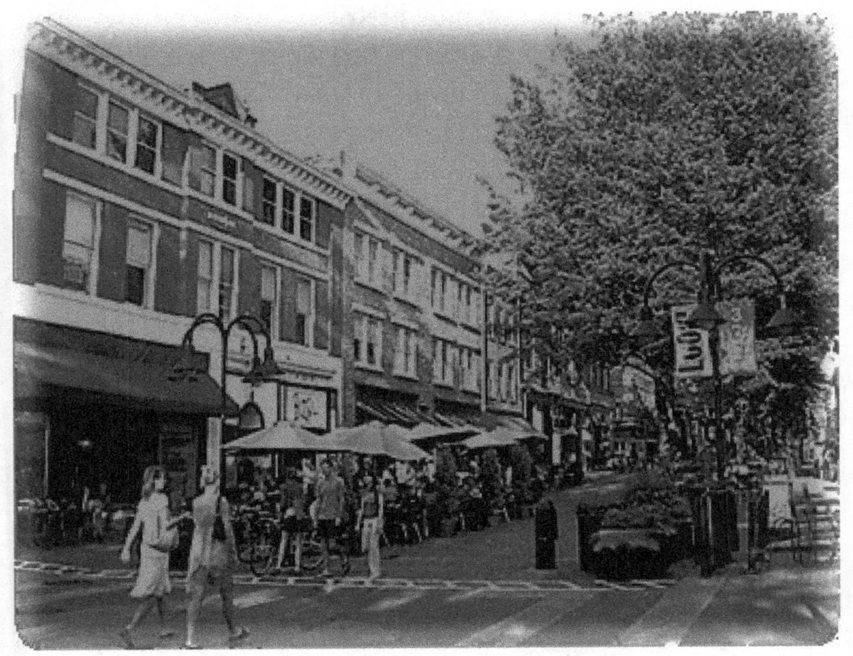

Try Thinking Inside The Box

Wash Hands, Wear Masks and Practice Social Distancing!

Most of us know the expression, "Try thinking out of the box." Certainly the Covid-19 Pandemic has challenged each of us to "think out of the box" as we have drastically changed the way we go about our daily lives. However, at this time we also need to learn to think "inside the box," both figuratively and literally.

The odds are poor, at best, that we have seen the last of the Covid-19 virus. There is a good chance we will see new spikes of the Covid-19 in new areas or in areas where people have let down their guard and have assumed the worst is over. Based upon past history of world pandemics there is a very good possibility that we may see a second wave in next winter and a smaller third wave a year later. I read this information in several documents and it made a definite impact on my thinking.

Each family is different...different sizes, different ages, and different stages. For sure, families are not a "one size fits all" proposition. This section of the book contains ideas for coping in a second wave, as well as information that may help families keep pandemic life in perspective.

First, Outside The Box

The Covid-19 Pandemic has forced all of us to slow down. It has forced us to reexamine our priorities and how we interact with others. The Pandemic affects the entire world. We are all under attack. Covid-19 is an equal opportunity virus. It doesn't separate people by class, race, religion, politics, or where we live. The entire world population faces this pandemic together.

As parents, we set the example for our children. We can each do our part: sheltering in place, wearing face masks, and washing our hands many times a day for 20 seconds. More importantly, our children see and learn how we treat other people. They see if we make frequent phone calls to family members, just to say hello and check to see if they need help. Our children see if we reach out and help elderly or people who may be high risk for the virus. Our children also see if we reach out and help our community get through the pandemic.

Indeed, we are the role models for our children. What we do, what we say, and how we behave towards others, especially during the Covid-19 Pandemic, is what our children in internalize and how they will approach their adult life. The Covid-19 Pandemic is a defining moment for our children's generation.

This is the time for parents to think out of box for the future of our children.

Second, Inside The Box

Most parts of this book are focused on school age children; elementary, junior high, and high school. Each level includes a wide variety of positive activities. Hopefully they have sparked new ideas for your family.

This section is about creating a Pandemic First Aid Kit. "What you say? What is a Pandemic First Aid Kit?"

As restrictions are slowly lifted, it will be easy for people to renew old habits and engage in very risky behaviors.

There will very likely be new spikes in Covid-19 across the country because some will think Covid-19 is over or that the Covid-19 virus has run its path and will fade away.

More important, a second wave of Covid-19 is very likely to hit hard during the 2020 fall and winter. A third, less deadly wave is likely in the fall and winter of 2021. Depending upon how successful scientists and researchers are in coming up with screening tests and vaccines, we could see schools stay closed or have to close again. My daughter is a vice principal at an elementary school. When I asked about how kids will social distance at school, she simply laughed at me and asked. “Can you imagine trying to keep twenty-five kindergarteners six feet apart? It would be like trying to herd cats.”

We were caught by surprise at the rapid growth of Covid-19 cases and the number of deaths that occurred in the first few weeks of the pandemic. The increase in number each day was staggering. Hence, we should not be surprised if there are more Covid-19 virus waves and the possibility of having to shelter in place again. Plan ahead now! One idea is for families to create Pandemic First Aid Kits.

A Pandemic First Aid Kit is a real thing. Looking back to the long shelter in place, what do you wish you had in the house that you did not have? Were there some basic items that would have made sheltering in place easier for your children? I have heard from several moms that they wish they had put together a little survival kit for each of their children. So, let’s start thinking about creating a Pandemic First Aid Kit.

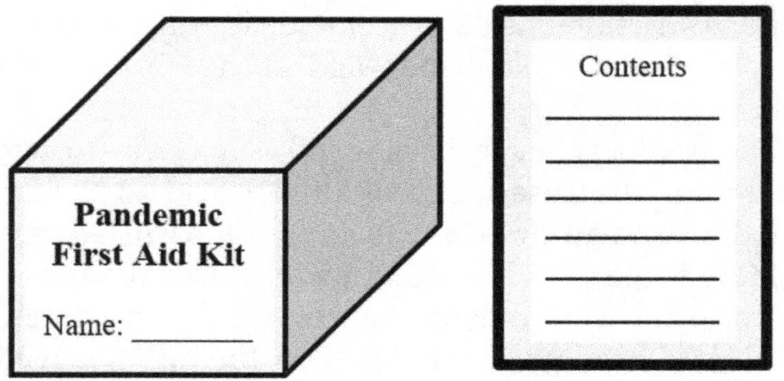

First off is a cardboard box – a banker’s box or larger. Hopefully it has a lid.

You may have several items on each list around the house – don't rebuy. It's also not necessary to put them in the kit. Just add them onto the list so you will not forget when you need to remember.

Mom First!

MOM FIRST!

MOM'S
PANDEMIC
KIT

FIRST AID

As a mom, what would you include in your own Pandemic First Aid Kit? What will make it easier to survive with your kids and husband? Place a few special items in your Pandemic First Aid Kit.

- Two of the largest dark chocolate bars available
- Two extra-large rolls of toilet paper – just for me!
- Two large bottles of hand sanitizer
- A box of face masks – just in case
- Pen, paper, envelopes and stamps
- Favorite soap, hand cream, and night cream
- A couple of good books or favorite magazines

- A favorite card or board game
- Two or more favorite music CDs.
- Items you need for your favorite hobby
- A personal calendar and personal phone book
- Stay connected with friends
- Favorite ways to relax
- The most important thing is: Plan now how to take care of you!

Pandemic First Aid Kits

Ideas for ages 3 – 7 (some beginning ideas, you will have better ones.)

- A couple of card games they like...Uno, Go Fish, etc.
- A couple of board games...Candy Land, etc.
- A couple of favorite books
- A new card game, board game, book at their level.
- Math or Sight Word Flash Cards
- Math, Language Arts, Science Workbooks (Teacher Supply Store)
- Easy Word Search Book
- Large roll of white shelf paper
- Washable colored markers or felt tip pens
- Box of large, thick crayons
- Box of sidewalk chalk
- Tablet of alphabet letters...to practice printing
- Large size Index Card...for making greeting cards
- Big roll of scotch tape

- Six primary grade sized pencils
- Scissors
- Paste or glue stick
- Old magazines with a lot of pictures to cut out
- Do a computer search for age appropriate games

Ideas for ages 8 – 12 (Beginning ideas, you and the kids will have better ones.)

- A couple of card games they like
- A couple of board games
- A couple of favorite books
- A new card game, board game, or book at their level.
- Math, Language Arts, Science Workbooks (Teacher Supply Store)
- Word Search Book
- Easy Cross Word Puzzle Book
- Large roll of white shelf paper
- Washable colored markers or felt tip pens
- Large box of crayons
- Easy learning to draw book
- Large size drawing pad
- Box of sidewalk chalk
- Large size Index Card...for making greeting cards
- Big roll of scotch tape
- Scissors

Ideas for ages 12+ (Some ideas, your kids will have better ones.)

- A couple of card games they like

- A couple of board games
- A new card game, board game, book
- Math, Language Arts, Science Workbooks (Teacher Supply Store)
- Word Search Book
- Word Puzzle Book
- Large roll of white shelf paper
- Washable colored markers or felt tip pens
- Large size Index Card...for making greeting cards
- Big roll of scotch tape
- Scissors

You may have a few things on each list already around the house. It's not necessary to put everything in the kit. Just add them to the list inside the lid so you will not forget when you need to remember.

It would be great if you did not ever need to use your Pandemic First Aid Kits. You can always save them for cold days during winter break or on hot days during summer vacation.

Pandemic Kit For Dad

A Pandemic First Aid Kit for myself. My first thought is a few bottles of... My next thought is a complete set of hair clippers. (I almost had to get a dog license during the last shelter in place.) How about a game that both my wife and I enjoy playing? I am also thinking about adding a game I would like to teach to my children. Let's include two good books that I have put off reading for the past couple of years. Finally, I will put a copy of my favorite saying into my kit.

NO ONE CAN DO EVERYTHING.
EVERYONE CAN DO SOMETHING.
WORKING TOGETHER,
WE ACCOMPLISH ABSOLUTELY
AMAZING THINGS!

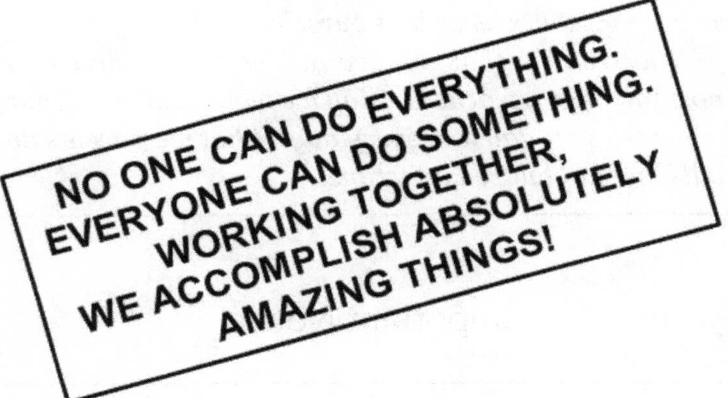

JUST REMEMBER

Remember that you matter,

your children matter, your family matters.

"Wash Hands! Wear Masks!

Practice Social Di-stancing!"

If you do not like wearing a mask, you are

really going to hate a ventilator.

Most of all, "Be Safe!"

Life Lesson: *This is the time people can find their better selves and model compassion, empathy and helping others especially for their children. We* *are all in this pandemic together. May we learn to see how we are alike and not so different. May we see the importance of being a part the greater community and caring for others as well as ourselves.*

The truth is that we are our children's first and most important teachers. May we teach and model our better selves today and every day. What we parents do will last our children a lifetime.

Important Notice

As the country reopens, be aware of what is happening with the Covid-19 virus in your local area. The number of active cases will be greater and on the rise in some areas and in some states. In other areas and states the cases of Covid-19 may be falling. With restrictions being eased and more and more stores reopening, be aware and cautious. Make decisions based upon local information. If you are going to err, err on the side of caution. Be safe and stay safe!

TRIBUTE

Graduate Together 2020

America Honors the High School Class of 2020

Five minutes after finishing this book, I sat down to watch **GRADUATE TOGETHER 2020** on television. While writing this book, I had never taken time to really think about the seniors of 2020. Many comments during Graduate Together 2020 could not help but touch my soul.

Every generation has a defining moment,

a collective experience. This is ours.

It is not what we lost. It is what we found.

When we get knocked down, we get up!

Impossible is nothing!

We will push forward!

We will fight like hell to create the future

we want.

The Class of 2020 is tied together forever and nothing will ever break our bond.

With enduring appreciation of the
Class of 2020, May 16, 2020

ABOUT THE AUTHOR

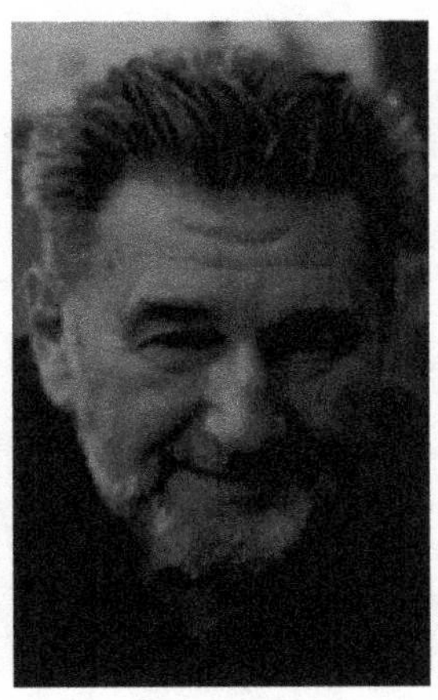

Meril Smith grew up at the end of World War II with children of migrant farm workers, children born in the Japanese internment camps, and children of day laborers and blue-collar workers. Poverty, recessions, and helping each other were all basic parts of surviving.

Living through the times of the Berlin Wall, the Salk polio vaccine, economic recessions, the space race, the development of Silicon Valley, and the Vietnam War fueled Meril's passion for understanding people and events. His training, life experience, and career provides an excellent backdrop for writing *Riding the Waves During A Pandemic*.